Understanding Social Work Practice in Mental Health

Understanding Social Work Practice in Mental Health

Vicki Coppock and Bob Dunn

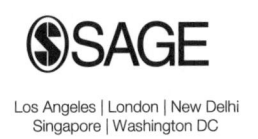

⑤SAGE

Los Angeles | London | New Delhi
Singapore | Washington DC

© Vicki Coppock and Bob Dunn 2010

First published 2010

Apart from any fair dealing for the purposes of research or private study, or criticism or review, as permitted under the Copyright, Designs and Patents Act 1988, this publication may be reproduced, stored or transmitted in any form, or by any means, only with the prior permission in writing of the publishers, or in the case of reprographic reproduction, in accordance with the terms of licences issued by the Copyright Licensing Agency. Enquiries concerning reproduction outside those terms should be sent to the publishers.

SAGE Publications Ltd
1 Oliver's Yard
55 City Road
London EC1Y 1SP

SAGE Publications Inc.
2455 Teller Road
Thousand Oaks, California 91320

SAGE Publications India Pvt Ltd
B 1/I 1 Mohan Cooperative Industrial Area
Mathura Road
New Delhi 110 044

SAGE Publications Asia-Pacific Pte Ltd
33 Pekin Street #02-01
Far East Square
Singapore 048763

Library of Congress Control Number: 2009924028

British Library Cataloguing in Publication data

A catalogue record for this book is available from the British Library

ISBN 978-1-4129-3504-3
ISBN 978-1-4129-3505-0 (pbk)

Typeset by C&M Digitals (P) Ltd, Chennai, India
Printed and bound in Great Britain by the MPG Books Group
Printed on paper from sustainable resources

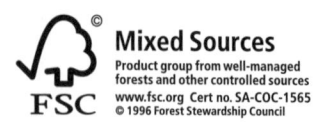

Mixed Sources
Product group from well-managed forests and other controlled sources
www.fsc.org Cert no. SA-COC-1565
© 1996 Forest Stewardship Council
FSC

CONTENTS

About the authors	vi
Introduction	1
1 Understanding mental health and mental distress	5
2 Thinking the present historically: the making of the modern mental health system	23
3 Care in the community: policy ideals and practice realities	39
4 Risk versus rights: the tensions in implementing mental health law	61
5 What works in promoting recovery? Evidence-based practice and the dynamics of power in mental health research	86
6 Challenging inequality and respecting diversity	106
7 Crossing cultures: interprofessional working in mental health	127
Conclusion	146
Bibliography	149
Index	165

ABOUT THE AUTHORS

Vicki Coppock is Reader in Social Work and Mental Health in the Department of Social and Psychological Sciences at Edge Hill University, Lancashire. She is also a qualified and experienced mental health social worker. She has a research and publications record in the critical analysis of theory, policy, legislation and professional practice in the field of mental health. Vicki is co-author of *Critical Perspectives on Mental Health* (Routledge, 2000) with John Hopton and had overall editorial responsibility for *Understanding Social Work Practice in Mental Health*.

Bob Dunn is Senior Lecturer also in the Department of Social and Psychological Sciences at Edge Hill University where he has taught for the last ten years. His teaching covers social work, childhood studies and youth justice. Some of Bob's previous responsibilities include working as a local authority Staff Development and Training Officer and running a unit for disturbed adolescents at the Cotswold Community. He has also researched deaths in prison, police and psychiatric custody.

INTRODUCTION

In the first decade of the twenty-first century mental health practitioners have witnessed unprecedented changes in mental health law and policy that have had profound consequences for their professional practice. In this book we explore the historical, theoretical and political contexts underpinning these changes and their impact on mental health practitioners and on users of mental health services and their carers. Many of the changes that have taken place (and are still taking place) relate to the emergence of new professional roles, skills and systems of service delivery that are no longer so clearly tied to traditional disciplinary lines. The traditional boundaries around 'who does what' in mental health care are being renegotiated and users of mental health services and their carers are increasingly influential in shaping the modern mental health system.

In this context it might then appear strange that this book should address itself to understanding *social work* practice in mental health. However, the focus on social work is deliberate and our defence of this rests in our belief in the central importance and distinctive contribution that social work makes in advancing a *social* model of mental health theory and practice that is highly valued by users of mental health services and their carers. Unlike many other mental health professions, social work has not always been very good at articulating precisely what it is that it brings to the field of mental health. In recent years this has started to change and, as we will discuss in this book, perhaps out of the necessity to ensure its survival, social work is reasserting its identity.

Understanding Social Work Practice in Mental Health will enable students of social work develop core knowledge, understanding, skills and values for professional social work practice in the mental health context. However, it is not an instruction manual on 'how to do mental health social work'. Rather, we firmly believe that it is only through a critical social scientific interrogation of the modern mental health system that students can learn to develop as critically reflective practitioners. Social workers are currently the only mental health practitioners with social science training. Whereas traditionally the emphasis in mental health education and training is on medical diagnosis, treatments and medication and mental health law, social work students are concerned with:

- developing an understanding of mental health theory, law, policy and practice as contested arenas
- developing a critical awareness of various theoretical and ideological perspectives that have contributed to knowledge about mental health and mental distress in multi-professional contexts

- developing an understanding of the complex moral and ethical dimensions underpinning mental health theory, law, policy and practice
- developing an understanding of, and way of working with, the personal and social consequences of inequality, discrimination, stigma and abuse
- learning to tolerate uncertainty and complexity in practice.

This book is deliberately designed to encourage students to critically examine the world of mental health theory, law, policy and practice from a variety of perspectives – those of users of mental health services, their carers and mental health professionals. To achieve this we use case studies, exercises and questions to stimulate debate and engage readers in critical reflection on key contemporary issues in mental health practice. Explicit links are made to academic and professional standards, codes of practice and frameworks for social work and mental health. Saying this, the book is not *exclusively* directed at students of mental health social work. The range of issues explored here should be of equal interest and relevance to other mental health practitioners – particularly given the strong drive in government policy towards interprofessional education, training and practice. Additionally, the book is designed to be of interest to anyone studying mental health and mental distress outside of the professional context.

In Chapter 1 we explore the contested nature of mental health and mental distress, introducing the different terminology, concepts and theories used in the field. This will include lay understandings of and attitudes towards mental distress in addition to professional perspectives, as both are significant in contemporary mental health practice. The power of language, images and representations of mental health and mental distress that circulate in society and contribute to the construction of the person in mental distress as 'other' is a key theme. Readers are invited to examine and reflect on their own personal attitudes to mental distress as a basis for understanding the stigma that is associated with receiving a mental health diagnosis. We outline and debate the relative contribution of medical and social models of mental health and illustrate the tensions between them in the context of how a person becomes a user of mental health services. We conclude with a discussion of the importance of developing a holistic, user-centred approach to mental health assessment.

In Chapter 2 we review the background to the modern mental health system with specific reference to the various historical perspectives on the emergence of British psychiatry and the development of formal institutionalized mental health care – from madhouses to asylums; from asylums to mental hospitals; and from hospitals to community mental health care. The origins and development of social work practice with the mentally distressed in this early period are also outlined and discussed.

Building on the discussion from the latter part of Chapter 2, Chapter 3 traces the implementation and further development of community care policy and practice for the mentally distressed from the early 1990s to the present. We begin by exploring what is meant by 'community care', acknowledging the role of 'informal carers' – that is care provided by relatives, friends, neighbours and volunteers. The implementation of the NHS and Community Care Act 1990 is subjected to critical evaluation and the role of the media in cultivating a climate of fear amongst the general public around community care for the mentally distressed is also explored. The chapter moves on to outline the 'modernization' policy reforms introduced by the New Labour government from the late 1990s onwards, including the *National Service Framework for Mental Health* (DH, 1999a) and the modern Care Programme Approach. The chapter concludes with a critical discussion around New Labour's 'personalization agenda' as it relates to those in mental distress.

Chapter 4 deals with the highly controversial subject of the compulsory detention of individuals identified as mentally disordered and the inherent tensions and conflicts faced by mental health practitioners when implementing mental health law. Indeed these tensions and conflicts have dominated the history of mental health legislation in England and Wales. The statutory context for modern mental health practice is explained, including the sectioning process and the roles of the various individuals and organizations related to it. The politics of compulsory detention and treatment are debated in the context of the burgeoning contemporary emphasis on managing risk in mental health practice. The chapter concludes with a discussion of the significance of human rights legislation in mental health practice and establishes some principles of good practice in implementing mental health law.

One of the most important consequences of the power of psychiatric theory is that it determines how people with mental health problems are responded to. Throughout the history of mental health care it has been possible to identify preferences in the approach to 'treatment'. However, there is an overriding unresolved tension between those psychiatric technologies that are primarily directed at the body and those which focus on the mind. In Chapter 5 we explore and critique some of the main contemporary approaches to treating mental distress – physical, psychological and social. Recent developments around the notion of 'recovery' in mental health care are discussed with particular emphasis on user-definitions of what this term means and how best to promote it. The chapter concludes with a critical discussion of evidence-based practice and the dynamics of power in mental health research. Crucially this will address the question of 'what counts as evidence and who decides'? It is argued that those in mental distress and their carers are 'experts by experience' and therefore user-focused and user-led approaches should be at the heart of mental health research and evaluation.

Drawing on Thompson's (2006) PCS (personal, cultural, structural) analysis, we begin Chapter 6 by theorizing the processes that produce and sustain inequalities, discrimination and oppression in the lives of people who use services. We then move on to explore how the dynamics of discrimination and inequality shape the lives of people in mental distress and their experiences of mental health services. Key diversity issues for mental health practitioners are highlighted including: class; race and ethnicity; gender; sexual orientation; disability; and age. The history of collective resistance to psychiatric oppression is acknowledged in an examination of the growth and impact of the mental health user movement. The chapter concludes with a discussion of the need for human rights based approaches to mental health care.

Chapter 7 provides an overview of the policy developments underpinning the move towards integrated services and interprofessional working in mental health, and critically analyses the implications of these for workforce development, education and training and service delivery. Messages from research studies evaluating interprofessional working in mental health are highlighted and the tensions between social work and health practitioners are explored. The chapter concludes with a discussion of the challenges currently facing social workers in integrated mental health teams and reasserts the distinctive contribution of social workers to high quality user- and carer-centred mental health care.

Finally, in the conclusion we revisit some of the central themes of the book and reassert the argument that critically reflective practice must be underpinned by a solid grounding in critical social science. We focus on what it means to be a critically reflective practitioner, emphasizing how the knowledge, skills and values of social work in particular are consistent with the expectations of what is required to meet the 'future vision' for mental health services (Future Vision Coalition, 2008).

1. UNDERSTANDING MENTAL HEALTH AND MENTAL DISTRESS

This chapter can be used to support the development of knowledge and skills in professional social work as follows:

National Occupational Standards for Social Work

Key Role 1: Prepare for and work with individuals, families, carers, groups and communities to assess their needs and circumstances

- Prepare for social work contact and involvement.

Key Role 3: Support individuals to represent their needs, views and circumstances

- Advocate with and on behalf of, individuals, families, carers, groups and communities.

Key Role 6: Demonstrate professional competence in social work practice

- Managing complex ethical issues, dilemmas and conflicts.

(TOPPS England, 2002)

Academic Standards for Social Work

Honours graduates in social work:

4.4 should be equipped to understand, and to work within, the context of contested debate about the nature, scope and purpose of social work, and be enabled to analyse, adapt to, manage and eventually to lead the processes of change.

4.6 must learn to:

- recognise and work with the powerful links between intrapersonal and interpersonal factors and the wider social, legal, economic, political and cultural context of people's lives
- understand the impact of injustice, social inequalities and oppressive social relations
- challenge constructively individual, institutional and structural discrimination.

4.7 should learn to become accountable, reflective, critical and evaluative which involves learning to:

- think critically about the complex social, political and cultural contexts in which social work is located.

5.1 should acquire, critically evaluate, apply and integrate knowledge and understanding in relation to:

5.1.1 Social work services, service users and carers

- the social processes (associated with, for example, poverty, migration, unemployment, poor health, disablement, lack of education and other sources of disadvantage) that lead to marginalisation, isolation and exclusion and their impact on the demand for social work services
- explanations of the links between definitional processes contributing to social differences (for example, social class, gender, ethnic differences, age, sexuality and religious belief) to the problems of inequality and differential need faced by service users
- the nature and validity of different definitions of, and explanations for, the characteristics and circumstances of service users and the services required by them, drawing on knowledge from research, practice experience, and from service users and carers.

5.1.4 Social work theory

- research-based concepts and critical explanations from social work theory and other disciplines that contribute to the knowledge base of social work, including their distinctive epistemological status and application to practice
- the relevance of sociological perspectives to understanding societal and structural influences on human behaviour at individual, group and community levels
- the relevance of psychological and physiological perspectives to understanding individual and social development and functioning
- models and methods of assessment, including factors underpinning the selection and testing of relevant information, the nature of professional judgement and the processes of risk assessment and decision-making.

5.5.3 should be able to analyse and synthesise information gathered for problem solving purposes to:

- assess the merits of contrasting theories, explanations, research, policies and procedures
- critically analyse and take account of the impact of inequality and discrimination in work with people in particular contexts and problem situations.

(QAA, 2008)

Understanding Mental Health and Mental Distress

Key themes in this chapter

- The scope and definitions of mental health and mental distress
- Examining personal attitudes towards mental distress
- The power of language, images and representations of mental health and mental distress
- Theorizing mental health – medical and social models
- Becoming a user of mental health services
- Developing an holistic, user-centred approach to mental health assessment.

INTRODUCTION

This chapter introduces the different terminology, concepts and theories used to describe and understand mental health and mental distress. This is an important starting point as it is vital that practitioners appreciate the diverse, often antagonistic, nature of the language, ideas and explanations that have evolved in this area over time. Pilgrim and Rogers (2005) and Parker et al. (1995) explain that what we know about mental health and mental distress has been influenced in two ways; first through popular culture (everyday language, popular fiction, painting, photography, songs, news and entertainment media) and secondly through professional discourses (psychiatry, psychology, social work and the law). These interact in complex ways producing a powerful fusion of common-sense and 'scientific' knowledge that can be difficult to unravel. Therefore this chapter also involves a critical analysis of the relationship between lay and professional knowledge in this field in order to understand the basis of contemporary mental health practice. The process of becoming a user of mental health services is subjected to critical examination, and in particular the process of mental health assessment. As you engage with the materials and exercises you will learn to appreciate that the knowledge base of mental health social work is far from straightforward. Social work practice in this field is inherently complicated, with assessments and interventions often fraught with controversy, tension and contradiction.

DEFINITIONS AND TERMINOLOGY

It is often argued that lay attitudes towards people in mental distress reflect a lack of understanding and knowledge (MIND, 2007a; Thornicroft et al., 2007). For example, surveys of the general public consistently show confusion about what mental distress actually is (DH, 2003a). However, this is not really surprising since there is significant disagreement amongst academics and professionals on this. Ways of understanding and defining mental health and mental distress are constantly changing in what is essentially a contested and dynamic arena. Finding a unified definition of what constitutes mental 'health' and mental 'illness' can be a frustrating exercise and something of a holy grail. For example, mental health can be defined either negatively, as 'the absence of objectively diagnosable disease' (WHO, 1946), or positively, as 'a state of well-being in which the individual realises his or her own abilities, can cope with the normal stresses of life, can work productively and fruitfully and is able to make a contribution to his or her community' (WHO, 2001a). The Mental Health Act 2007 introduced a single definition of 'mental disorder' as 'any disorder or disability of the mind'.

The confusion and controversy surrounding mental distress is also clearly reflected in the diverse terminology used in the field – mental health; mental illness; mental disorder; mental health problem; mental distress. Although these terms are often used interchangeably, they actually derive from quite different philosophical, theoretical and ideological perspectives. That is, the terminology used to describe a person's mental health status is grounded in the particular approach to understanding mental health subscribed to by the particular individual, group or organization using the term. So for example, broadly speaking, traditional mainstream psychological or psychiatric literature will opt for the terms mental illness and/or mental disorder in keeping with a psycho-*medical* paradigm, while critical social scientific or user-centred literature tends towards the terms mental health problem or mental distress reflecting a psycho-*social* paradigm. These contrasting models of mental health are discussed later in this chapter.

In this book we have shown a conscious preference for the term 'mental distress', as this most closely reflects both our value position in relation to people who use mental health services and our critical social scientific approach to the subject. Occasionally we use the terms mental illness and/or mental disorder where we feel it is important to remain consistent with the original context in which the term is used (for example, when discussing official definitions used in mental health law or policy), but when doing so we indicate the contested nature of that term through the use of single inverted commas – as in 'mental illness'.

EXAMINING OUR ATTITUDES TO MENTAL DISTRESS

From the outset it is important to acknowledge and reflect on our own *individual* feelings, attitudes and understanding of mental health and mental distress. Neil Thompson (2006) explains how practitioners need to be aware that they do not practise in a moral and political vacuum. His 'PCS' analysis (Figure 1.1) is an extremely useful tool in assisting practitioners to develop their understanding of the relationship between wider society, popular culture and individual attitudes.

Thompson (2006) reminds us that the way we come to understand and behave towards the world around us, and the people within it, is primarily shaped by the culture in which we live. As essentially subjective beings, health and social care professionals are no less immune to the influence of prejudicial ideas, attitudes and behaviours. Acknowledging this fact is an important first step towards becoming a

Understanding Mental Health and Mental Distress

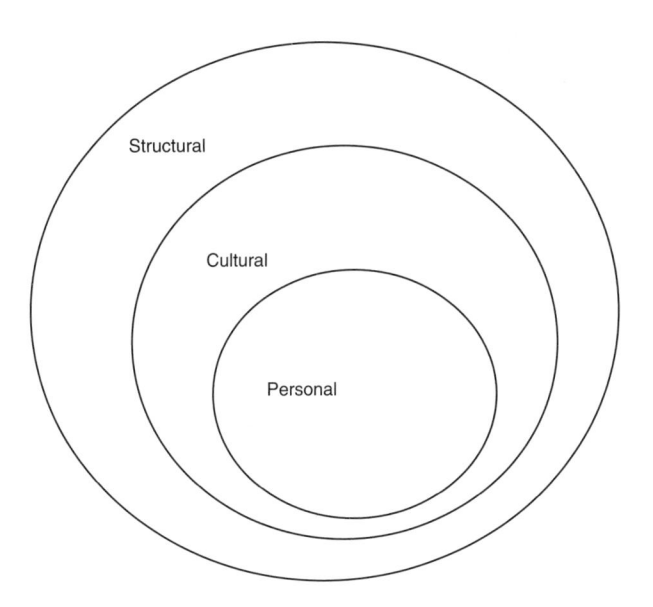

[Diagram: Three concentric circles labelled, from outer to inner: Structural, Cultural, Personal]

Figure 1.1 Thompson's (2006) PCS Analysis

critically self-aware practitioner, capable of identifying and then redressing any personal discriminatory beliefs and practices. We will return to Thompson's analysis and discuss its application to anti-oppressive social work practice in mental health more fully in Chapter 6.

Reflection exercise

How do *you* feel about people in mental distress? Write down as many words as you can to describe your feelings. Be honest with yourself!

It is highly likely that somewhere on your list the words 'fear' and 'sympathy' will have appeared, or at least words that convey similar meanings. These are extremely common emotional reactions that people have to those in mental distress. The diverse, complex and extraordinary ways in which mental distress is manifest in human beings can be disturbing, and at times frightening, for those experiencing it, those close to them and those working with them. The UK Department of Health has conducted regular surveys of people's attitudes to mental distress since 1993 and these two themes have featured prominently and consistently in people's responses. Moreover, although fear and sympathy might initially appear to reflect quite different value positions, people often express sympathy and concern for the mentally distressed while simultaneously expressing support for actions that effectively stigmatize and exclude them from the rest of society. This reveals how attitudes towards people with mental health problems are extremely complex and often contradictory.

> ### Reflection exercise
>
> How do you feel about *your own* mental health? Reflecting on your own life experiences, write down some words or phrases to describe your mental health at significant times. Again, be honest with yourself!

Official statistics indicate that one in six people might experience a mental health problem during their lifetime (Singleton et al., 2001). However, in research conducted by the Department of Health (DH, 2003a), 49 per cent of people reported knowing someone who had experienced mental distress, while only seven per cent admitted that they had experienced mental distress themselves. Similarly, in a MORI survey in 1995, 23 per cent of respondents said that if they were receiving psychiatric treatment they would be reluctant or unwilling to admit this to their friends:

> It often seems a good idea to keep quiet about my mental distress. Yet when I am asked why I don't drink or why I took a year out from university, it would be nice to say, 'I was ill with schizophrenia' or 'I take medication for schizophrenia' without fear of a negative reaction. (Service user, cited in MIND, 2007a)

This suggests that although mental distress is statistically a common experience and part of everyday human existence, we have a tendency to want to distance ourselves from it – to see it as something far removed from us. Furthermore, this seems to confirm the existence of a deep-seated fear of, or taboo around, mental distress in our society: 'I found that people do one of two things. They look at you in one of two ways. Some look ashamed and furtive because … I suppose everyone talks, and everyone is afraid of madness'. (Nicola Pagett, from *Diamonds Behind My Eyes*, cited in MIND, 2003a).

There is plenty of historical and cross-cultural evidence to show how the mentally distressed have been feared and excluded from mainstream society. In *Madness and Civilisation* Foucault tells us how:

> Suddenly, in a few years in the middle of the eighteenth century, a fear arose – a fear formulated in medical terms but animated, basically, by a moral myth … the fear of madness grew at the same time as the dread of unreason: and thereby the two forms of obsession, leaning upon each other, continued to reinforce each other. (1967: 192–200)

Denise Jodelet's (1991) longitudinal research in rural France illustrates the persistence of alienating and exclusionary practices towards the mentally distressed despite their deinstitutionalization and official integration into the community. The rhetorical acceptance of these people into the community was not matched by the reality of their status within it – their 'otherness' dictated that they only had a token place in the real world. Similar evidence has emerged from research into the social networks of mentally distressed people discharged into the community in the UK (Repper et al., 1997; Taylor 1994/95) and Ireland (Prior, 1993).

Recent evidence suggests that public attitudes may actually be worsening. In 2007, the Department of Health's *Attitudes to Mental Illness* survey found an increase in prejudice across a wide variety of indicators, including: not wanting to live next door to someone diagnosed with mental distress; not believing that the mentally distressed have the same right to a job as anyone else; and believing that they are prone to violence (TNS, 2007). This suggests that very powerful ideological forces are present and that these are in tension with, if not resistant to, progressive social and political developments aimed at improving the lives of the mentally distressed in society. Therefore, our reluctance to admit to experiencing mental health problems in contemporary society is not simply to do with the existential fear of 'otherness' – it is as much to do with the *material* consequences of 'exposure' in the form of inequality, discrimination and oppression (Mental Health Media, 2008). As Sayce observes, 'increasing social inequality … impacts on people with mental health problems both because social exclusion itself creates distress and because those who are disadvantaged by the social status of the 'mental patient' become caught up in punitive, excluding policies and public moods' (2000: 41). We discuss the relationship between mental distress, inequality, discrimination and oppression more fully in Chapter 6.

IMAGES AND REPRESENTATIONS OF MENTAL DISTRESS

Research has pointed to the important role played by the news and entertainment media in constructing negative attitudes towards people in mental distress (Clarke, 2004; CSIP/Shift, 2006; Philo, 1996).

Group reflection exercise

Spend a week analysing the content of newspapers, magazines, radio, television and film, collecting examples of the use of imagery and language relating to mental health/mental distress. Share your findings with a small group of fellow students and discuss the following questions:

How do you think such images/language affect people in mental distress? How can mental health practitioners contribute to promoting a positive image of users of mental health services?

It is highly likely that your examples will include stereotypical images of the mentally distressed as violent, unpredictable and dangerous. Research demonstrates that these are particularly dominant themes, often wildly exaggerated (Clarke, 2004; CSIP/ Shift, 2006; Laurence, 2003; Philo, 1996). Such representations are in stark contrast to the research evidence that demonstrates how people with mental health problems are more likely to be victims than perpetrators of violence (Monahan, 1992; Taylor and Gunn, 1999). People in mental distress are three times more likely to experience harassment (ranging from verbal abuse to violent attacks) in their local community than the general population (Berzins et al., 2003; National Schizophrenia Fellowship Scotland, 2001). A participant in the MIND survey *Creating Accepting Communities* (Dunn, 1999) reported that he had been abused in the street; his house broken into twelve times and a knife put through the door. He wryly observed how, according to the media, he is supposed to be the one who is nasty and violent.

Philo (1996) explains that media representations are a very powerful influence on beliefs about the nature of mental distress and this often overrides people's personal experience – something which is very unusual in media research: 'A friend of many years, responding to media reports of killings by ex-psychiatric patients, said that psychiatric patients should all be locked up' (service user, cited in MIND, 2003a).

The examples you have noted are also likely to include the use of pejorative terminology associated with mental health such as 'psycho', 'schizo', 'loony' and 'nutter'. These terms are often used in conversations not directly relating to a person or persons with mental health problems – perhaps being used as a form of interpersonal abuse, insult or joke. This indicates how such pejorative terminology is deeply embedded in our vocabularies and how negative images of people in mental distress are partly constructed through the ordinary everyday language we use to talk about mental health. Some argue that there is no harm in such language and that to make a fuss about it is simply political correctness. However, many researchers, mental health professionals, service users and carers have written about the power of language in stigmatizing mental health patients (see for example Read and Baker, 1996). Pejorative language is oppressive because it dehumanizes the person: 'Mentioning the name of my illness makes people feel as though you're Norman Bates' (service user, cited in MIND, 2003a).

The MIND survey *Counting the Cost* (Baker and MacPherson, 2000) analysed the effects of media portrayals on the lives of people with mental distress. Half of those who took part in the survey said that media coverage had a negative effect on their mental health:

- 34 per cent reported feeling more anxious or depressed
- 24 per cent had experienced hostility from their neighbours as a result of media reports
- 33 per cent felt reluctant to apply for jobs or to volunteer
- 37 per cent said their families or friends reacted differently to them because of recent media coverage.

One of the obvious consequences of negative stereotyping is that people avoid seeking help for their mental distress for fear of the stigma that follows (Read and Baker, 1996). Negative images and stereotypes are so pervasive and damaging that national and international campaigns and programmes have been developed to reduce the stigma associated with mental distress. Some of these include the Care Services Improvement Partnership (CSIP) five-year initiative, *Shift* (2004–09) (www.shift.org.uk); the Mental Health Media, MIND, Rethink and Institute of Psychiatry campaign, *Time to Change* (previously *Moving People*) (2007–12) www.time-to-change.org.uk); the campaign by an alliance of five Scottish mental health organizations, *See Me* (2002–ongoing) (www.seemescotland.org.uk); the World Psychiatric Association campaign, *Open the Doors* (1996–ongoing) (www.wpanet.org/programs/opendoors-schizo.shtml); the Department of Health campaign, *Mind Out for Mental Health* (2001–04); the Royal College of Psychiatrists campaign, *Changing Minds* (1998–2003); and the MIND campaign, *Creating Accepting Communities* (1998–99). In the Moving People (2008) survey, *Stigma Shout,* 87 per cent of service users reported actual or anticipated stigma and/or discrimination.

Sartorious informs us that 'the stigma attached to mental illness, and to the people who have it, is a major obstacle to better care and to the improvement of the quality of their lives' (2002: 1470). Therefore it is essential that mental health practitioners and policy-makers challenge negative, damaging language, representations and attitudes in order to develop non-stigmatizing, accessible mental health care. Ironically, however, there is evidence to suggest that mental health professionals and mental health services may actually contribute to the stigmatization of people in mental distress – both through the diagnostic labelling process and in the way that treatments and services have traditionally been provided (Angermeyer and Matschinger, 2003; Sartorious, 2002). Sartorious (2002) illustrates how diagnostic labels can be an obvious source of stigmatization. While they might be useful in general medicine as a means of shorthand communication about a person's physical condition, their relevance and/or appropriateness in the mental health field has been questioned. Moreover, mistakes in psychiatric diagnosis can have devastating consequences – for example, the case of Kay Sheldon (cited in Double, 2001) who was forced to make a claim for medical negligence against her Health Authority after being misdiagnosed and treated for schizophrenia. The critical psychiatrist Pat Bracken highlights another downside to diagnosis and the medical framing of distress:

> It can cover up as well as illuminate the reasons for our pain and suffering. It is often presented to patients as 'the truth' of their condition and serves to silence other possibilities. Psychiatric diagnosis is often little more than a simplification of a complex reality and by formulating an individual's experiences in terms of pathology it can be profoundly disempowering and stigmatising. (2002: 27)

It seems astonishing that in the round table discussions on mental health during the 54th World Health Assembly it had to be conceded that 'most importantly, stigmatization, by all health professionals including mental health workers needed to be overcome' (WHO, 2001b). In the UK context, a Mental Health Foundation survey (2000) found that 44 per cent of respondents had experienced discrimination from their GPs, while 32 per cent had experienced discrimination from health care professionals other than GPs. Prominent among them were:

- nurses and other hospital staff on both general and psychiatric wards
- psychiatrists and consultants
- emergency staff, particularly in A&E departments in response to self-harm
- community and social services, such as CPNs and social workers.

Similarly, in research by Thornicroft (2006) two-thirds of service users identified the attitudes and behaviours of GPs and other health professionals as stigmatizing. Incidents reported included being deliberately punished by staff or treated with a lack of respect. Other first-hand accounts of people who use mental health services reveal a disturbing picture of stigmatizing and oppressive treatment as illustrated in the following quotations:

> Many mental health staff seem to embody the same stigma and discrimination that we might meet anywhere in society. Some staff treat us as if we are bad rather than mad, or talk to us as if we are naughty children.
>
> I have observed or experienced so many occasions where staff are clearly making a situation worse by shouting at people, or threatening people ... it only leads to further humiliation and shame for us. How hard is it to maintain any kind of self-esteem in the face of this?
>
> For over 12 years I have been a service user and have encountered an enormous amount of prejudice and total disregard for my feelings and intellect by the medical profession. I am a real life person with thoughts and feelings.
>
> What most frustrates me is being treated like a dangerous animal .... The only violence in my 14 years of contact has been perpetrated by staff on me: once as I came down a flight of stairs I was jumped, my arms pinned behind my back, and my head and chest over the banister and then being 'restrained', prone on the floor with four nurses pinning me down and two deliberately inflicting pain because I dared to want to sit in the garden.
> (Selection of service user accounts, cited in The *Guardian*, 18 October 2006)

Chaplin (2000) draws attention to other aspects of psychiatric practice that maintain the stigma of mental distress – for example, the highly visible presence of medical, social work and police services in compulsory Mental Health Act assessments, and the overt physical side-effects of medications prescribed by psychiatrists (such as drooling and involuntary movements) that can make individuals appear socially undesirable. Similarly, McKay notes the stigmatizing effects of advertisements for psychiatric drugs that appear in medical journals:

> How can we expect the general public to have a rational and informed approach to people with schizophrenia when learned journals accept advertisements that promote a product through negative stereotyping? Perhaps our willingness to allow this to happen is in accord with work in the field, which suggests that health professionals may have even more negative attitudes to mental disorder than the general public. (2000: 467)

THEORIZING MENTAL HEALTH – MEDICAL AND SOCIAL MODELS

In Western societies mental distress is almost universally understood as a belief that there is a disturbance in one or more areas of human functioning – thoughts, feelings and behaviours. Nevertheless, explanations for mental distress are a fiercely contested and debated area. Theories about the causes of mental distress vary between, and to some extent within, the various disciplines concerned with the field of mental health, though most conform to what is termed the medical or disease model. The medical model emerged from the mid-nineteenth century onwards, shifting earlier moral or religious frameworks of explanation for mental distress towards an illness framework. Psychiatry consolidated itself in the twentieth century through its assimilation with medicine, and the concept of 'mental illness' evolved as a generic term embracing a diversity of behaviours and phenomena. The modern day language and practice of mental health mimics that of the medical sciences in so far as it involves: the *observation* of human emotions and behaviour; the *identification* of pathological 'symptoms'; the *diagnosis* of 'disorders' or 'illnesses' and the prescription of appropriate *treatment* for these.

The medical model approach is underpinned by the belief that mental health diagnosis simply involves the accurate naming of an objective disease process (Bracken and Thomas, 2000). The *Diagnostic and Statistical Manual of Mental Disorders* (DSM), published by the American Psychiatric Association (2000), is the system used most often by psychiatrists in diagnosing mental disorders. The *International Statistical Classification of Diseases and Related Problems* (ICD) is a less widely used system published by the World Health Organization (1992). Both systems assume medical concepts and terminology and outline categorical disorders that can be diagnosed by set lists of criteria. The DSM has been revised five times since its inception in 1952. It was initially developed to create a standardized taxonomy that would enhance effective communication between psychiatrists to facilitate mental health research, diagnosis and treatment. The most recent version of the DSM is the DSM-IV-TR published in 2000.

Ostensibly, through the development of these formal diagnostic and classification systems, the medical model appears to provide practitioners with answers and certainties, but this can be a misleading assumption. Although they are modelled on the scientific paradigm, research has demonstrated that classification and diagnostic systems in the mental health field do not necessarily produce objective professional judgements. The process relies heavily on the interpretation of human emotions and behaviour, with diagnosis clearly capable of being influenced by subjective attitudes and beliefs (Double, 2002; Kirk and Kutchins, 1999). Double reminds us that 'psychiatrists do not want to admit the uncertainty that there is around diagnosis. One only needs to attend a psychiatric case conference to realise that diagnosis is not an exact science. Many different opinions will be expressed' (2001: 42).

The experience of learning to diagnose 'mental illness' is also influenced by the social, cultural and political contexts in which psychiatric training takes place, with a distinctly patriarchal, Western world-view dominating contemporary theory and practice

(Fernando, 2002; Loring and Powell, 1988). Similarly psychiatric knowledge itself is constantly under negotiation and changes over time. The contents of the DSM are determined through a process of periodic review and consultation by a panel of 'expert' psychiatrists. The number of classified disorders has grown significantly since the first edition (DSM-I) was published in 1952. From an initial list of some 128 disorders, the list had grown to 227 by the time DSM-III was published in 1980 and now stands at 374 in DSM-IV-TR (American Psychiatric Association, 2000). Some disorders have 'disappeared' altogether (most notably the de-classification of homosexuality as a mental disorder by a vote of the American Psychiatric Association in 1973 after a concerted campaign by gay activists) while new ones have apparently been 'discovered' (for example the introduction of 'religious or spiritual problem' in DSM-IV in 1994).

It is this uncertainty that has exposed psychiatry and the medical model in particular, to challenges to its authority. Throughout its history psychiatry has experienced dissent from within and outside the profession from those who contest the validity of the medical model of mental distress. Sociologists and dissident clinicians have argued that the emotions and behaviours that psychiatrists call 'symptoms' and 'illnesses' should not be considered pathological medical phenomena but meaningful 'problems of living' – manifestations of the social and political forces that shape the lives of human beings (see Foucault, 1967; Laing, 1959; Scheff, 1966; Szasz, 1961). The process by which people are categorized and labelled as 'mentally ill' is understood here as essentially *social* rather than medical – a means of pathologizing emotions and behaviours that society has deemed unacceptable. It is suggested that while the experience of mental distress is *real*, mental health problems are not, in fact, entities. It is misleading that the medical model speaks of them as though they are.

Furthermore, critics argue that formal psychiatric classification and diagnostic systems are subject to the limitations of the methods used to create them; 'psychiatric diagnosis is not dissimilar to astrology: both systems attempt to tell us something about people and to predict what will happen to them in the future, and both fail miserably' (Bentall, 2004: 21).

In practice, patients frequently fail to 'fit' into a particular category or, conversely, may fall into several. The categorical 'present or absent' approach to diagnosis encourages a polarized understanding of mental health rather than one which recognizes human experience as richly diverse and fluid, and better represented as a continuum. More significant, perhaps, is the criticism that rigid adherence to formal classification and diagnostic systems 'encourages unthinking practice and an impersonal approach' (Double, 2001: 43). Diagnosis, when used as a form of measurement, can easily overlook the uniqueness of individuals and important information can be lost that might otherwise help practitioners to fully understand the reason for the person's mental distress. As Poole acknowledges:

> Psychiatric diagnosis is like a map reference. It tells you the general type of psychological terrain the patient is in; it tells you how this patient's disorder relates to other disorders, physical and mental. It conveys some limited predictive information, and a general indication of the types of intervention that might be helpful. However, just as a map reference cannot tell you the appearance of the landscape, similarly a psychiatric diagnosis

does not tell you what the person is like, how s/he will behave and the nature of any risks s/he faces. These matters have to be assessed individually on the basis of knowledge of the person. (2006: 134)

By contrast, the social model of mental distress privileges explanations that focus on independent life events that trigger breakdown (such as isolation, violence, bereavement and loss) and on social forces linked to: class (poverty and unemployment); race and ethnicity (racism); gender and sexuality (sexism and homophobia); age (ageism); and disability (disablism) that precipitate mental distress, recognizing that mental distress can be linked to issues of powerlessness, inequality and oppression (these issues are discussed more fully in Chapter 6).

In a national survey undertaken by MIND in 1990 mental health service users reported what it felt like to be on the receiving end of services (Rogers et al., 1993). Most saw their difficulties as rooted in the context of their life experiences rather than as symptoms of an illness. The responses of mental health professionals in primary and specialist settings were experienced as far too narrow and failed to engage with the priorities of service users. By contrast, the services that were valued were those that were in harmony with people's normal living arrangements, as well as services that engaged with issues related to housing, income, employment, isolation, relationships and meaningful occupation. The researchers concluded that mental health service users' needs are best framed broadly in personal and social rather than medical terms.

Advocates of the social model would argue that the medical model, on its own, is not sufficient to underpin policy and practice in mental health. The social model expands our understanding of mental distress beyond the narrow approach of just treating symptoms and provides frameworks that may be useful in giving meaning to the experiences of people in mental distress and in enabling and supporting their recovery (Tew, 2003). This does not necessarily imply an anti-psychiatry or anti-medication approach. Rather it is a model that refuses to privilege the medical model and pushes for the endorsement of a range of different perspectives on mental health (Bracken and Smyth, 2006). The next section explores further some of the essential differences between the medical and social models of mental distress with specific reference to the process of mental health assessment.

BECOMING A USER OF MENTAL HEALTH SERVICES: THE ASSESSMENT PROCESS

All assessments of mental health depend on theories about what constitute 'normal' thoughts, feelings and behaviours and how these can be distinguished from 'disordered' thoughts, feelings and behaviours. Nevertheless, as we have already established, the process of becoming a mental health service user begins well in advance of any direct contact with mental health professionals and is not solely influenced by formal professional judgements of what constitutes 'normality' and 'abnormality'. Other people (partners, parents and friends) will have already formed lay judgements about the person's mental state prior to any formal examination by a psychiatrist. Indeed, often what triggers contact with mental health services in the first instance is a third party's observation and/or concern that the person's mood or behaviour has changed, becoming 'odd' or 'out of character' (as in the case study of Brian below).

De Swaan (1990) explains that the medical model of mental health is so firmly established in Western culture that we have all become 'proto-patients' and 'proto-professionals' – constantly monitoring and interpreting our own emotional and behavioural states, and those of others, in distinctly medical terms. Similarly, Pilgrim and Rogers (2005) talk about a cultural consensus between professionals and the general public around the conceptualization and management of mental distress. Sociologists (Goffman, 1961; Scheff, 1966) have argued that lay diagnosis is the first step in establishing the person in mental distress as 'other' or 'outsider'. Subsequently, through formal psychiatric diagnosis, that person then acquires the identity of 'mental patient'.

The mental state examination is the first formal stage in the process of psychiatric assessment and diagnosis. This is undertaken by a medical doctor (who is usually also a psychiatrist) using the standardized 'tools' available to her/him. This process is accompanied by a multidisciplinary investigation of the person's psychiatric and social history drawn from discussions with the individual, and his or her family and friends. Two points need to be noted here. First, while mental health practitioners do have very specific duties, powers and responsibilities under the Mental Health Act 1983 (amended by the Mental Health Act 2007) to assess a person for whom compulsory admission to hospital may be required, mental health assessments are not restricted to the compulsory context. (A full discussion of the process of compulsory assessment under mental health legislation is provided in Chapter 4). Compulsory assessments make up only a small part of the work of community mental health teams. Routine multidisciplinary mental health assessments occur in a variety of other circumstances, most frequently in the context of needs-led assessments under the provisions of The NHS and Community Care Act 1990. Secondly, it is important to note that carers of those in mental distress also have the statutory right to an assessment of *their* needs alongside the assessment of those of the mental health service user, under the provisions of The Carers (Recognition and Services) Act 1995.

Case study

Brian Smith, aged 19, lives at home with his parents. He has suddenly become very reluctant to get up in the morning to go to university. He has become less talkative in recent weeks and spends most of his time in his bedroom, preferring his own company. Brian socializes less than he used to, refusing invitations to go out with friends. He shows little care for his appearance or personal hygiene. Brian's behaviour is now causing his parents serious concern and they have sought help from their family GP. The GP has asked the local mental health support team to visit the family home.

What steps need to be taken to ensure a thorough and accurate assessment of Brian's situation?

Explore the various theoretical models available to the team that might help them to (i) understand Brian's behaviour and (ii) assess Brian's situation.

Discussion: Case Study

As Bracken and Smyth point out, 'for professionals who are trained to see the world through "medical model" spectacles ... questions to do with meanings, relationships and values ... are understood to be secondary concerns' (*Irish Times*, 29 December 2006). If the practitioners in the team approach Brian's case from the perspective of the medical model of mental health their attention is likely to focus heavily on Brian himself. However in this context a focus at the level of the individual does not equate with being 'user-centred'. Quite the contrary, it relates to the assumption that 'the problem' primarily lies *within* the individual. Therefore the assessment process is heavily oriented towards the *form* of the distress rather than the *content* and *context* of the distressing experience. This can lead to the subordination or even denial of the individual's account and the privileging of 'expert' knowledge or explanations that focus on individual (invariably biological) pathology and which inevitably lead to individualized (usually pharmacological) treatment responses.

Furthermore, an overly medicalized model of assessment in mental health practice can reinforce assumptions about the risks posed *by* the mentally distressed – either to themselves or others – simply by virtue of their 'illness' or 'disorder'. Such an approach detracts from a full understanding of other dimensions of risk including social factors such as unemployment, poverty and domestic abuse and particularly the risks posed by the mental health system *to* the mentally distressed (Pilgrim and Rogers, 1996).

The social model approach to mental health assessment is informed by an understanding that 'making a judgement and assessment about another person inevitably involves values as well as facts' (Double, 2001: 42). This compels the practitioner to look beyond the level of the individual, to the wider context within which the individual, his/her immediate family/friends and the practitioner/mental health service are located. The need for a holistic approach to assessment is reflected in the *National Service Framework for Mental Health* (DH, 1999a).

Using Thompson's PCS analysis (see Figure 1.1, p. 9), we understand that Brian, his family and the mental health team do not exist in a 'bubble' – the social, political, economic and cultural forces that surround them influence both Brian's 'personhood' and how his family and mental health practitioners 'see' and make sense of his situation. Tew explains how social models 'explore the ways in which mental distress may be understood as, in part, a response to problematic life experiences' (2005: 20). In this context, Brian's mental distress may be understood as 'the internalisation or acting out of stressful experiences' or the development of 'a coping or survival strategy' rather than some internal 'illness' or 'disorder' (2005: 20). Therefore a full understanding of Brian's thoughts, emotions and behaviour will require an integration of *all* dimensions of his lived experience. As Double argues, 'what matters in assessment ... is an understanding of the patient as a person' (2001: 43).

A holistic approach to mental health assessment also requires critical self-awareness on the part of all those practitioners involved, acknowledging power differentials and how personal and agency values and perspectives influence the assessment process. A social model approach to mental health assessment acknowledges the validity of Brian's own account of his distress – as an 'expert by experience'. The need for people who use mental health services and their carers to be listened to and have their views taken seriously is a consistent theme in research literature (Beresford, 2007a; Rogers et al., 1993; Sayce, 2000).

This implies the need for a *partnership* approach to assessment – such an approach is consistent with a genuinely user-centred, empowering practice. A holistic approach to mental health assessment moves practitioners beyond the inherently stigmatizing medical model that imposes distinctions between 'normal' people and those suffering distress, or that tends to define the totality of a person in terms of their 'pathology' (Tew, 2002). As Tew argues, 'there is no room for "us" and "them" thinking that can divide service users from carers or practitioners' (cited in SPN, 2003a: 2).

Social workers are ideally situated to promote the social model approach to mental health assessment:

> Social work brings something distinctive to mental health. Articulating it is more difficult. It is a constellation of values, commitment to social justice and partnership with users and carers. Social workers practised social inclusion before the term had been invented. Above all in mental health, it challenges the traditional medical model which does not fully acknowledge the patient or client as best informed about their needs. (Bamford, 2006)

The distinctive contribution of social work to interdisciplinary working in mental health

Social work perspectives and knowledge base

Social work is about change. Social workers try to improve the circumstances of people who are vulnerable or face social exclusion both by building on their personal strengths and by changing the social circumstances which have contributed to their mental distress. This means that they take a community as well as an individual perspective. They are committed to principles of self-determination and of helping people to overcome discrimination and other barriers to achieving their potential.

The social work knowledge base brings together a range of social science perspectives, linked to an understanding of law and social policy as it affects users of social care services and their families or informal carers. Seeing the person in their social context, practitioners apply social models of mental health, with an emphasis on how personal and family relationships, cultural needs, housing, work and social networks may be integral to recovery.

Social work has particular expertise in relation to the social and environmental factors that contribute to mental distress through the life course. This includes the impact of abuse and stigma on personal development.

The profession is characterised by a strong tradition of critical questioning, reflection and challenge within a multi-disciplinary context.

Essential shared capabilities

Social work has long provided a key and integral contribution to mental health services. Social work values, skills and knowledge are closely aligned with the 'Ten Essential Shared Capabilities' Framework for mental health practice and emphasise empowerment, challenging inequalities and working in partnership with service users and carers to support recovery.

Distinctive practice capabilities of social workers

- Assessing complex situations, taking account of an individual's strengths, aspirations, and vulnerabilities within a context of their personal and family relationships, cultural needs, social and environmental stressors and connections within the community.
- Working alongside service users to promote their social inclusion – mobilizing a range of community resources, networks, and statutory and voluntary services.
- Balancing legal and human rights and issues of risk and safety – achieving the least restrictive alternative within statutory roles and responsibilities, while offering protection to those who may be at risk of exploitation or harm.
- Working with family and informal carers to support an individual's journey to recovery
- Identifying and working with the personal and social consequences of discrimination, stigma and abuse
- Seeking changes in the social and environmental context which will promote recovery.

(NWW4SW Sub Group, in SWAP/MHHE, 2007: 10)

The Social Perspectives Network for Modern Mental Health (SPN, 2003b) identifies a number of barriers to achieving user-centred practice including:

- the consistent undervaluing of users' perspectives
- the failure to acknowledge diversity
- the lack of attention to the complexity of people's experiences of mental distress
- the entrenchment of the narrow medical model.

Conversely, there are some key principles for achieving user-centred practice including:

- *Empowerment* – working with service users, not doing things to them; avoiding paternalism
- *Partnership* – seeing service users as 'experts by experience' – accepting the right of service users to define their own experience and to find their own solutions – not a 'professionals know best' attitude
- *Empathic approach* – a willingness to look at situations through the eyes of service users
- *Genuine involvement* – of service users and carers in the design and delivery of services.

These are central principles for practice that will feature prominently throughout this book.

CHAPTER SUMMARY

In this first chapter we have begun to unravel the different terminology, images and representations, concepts and theories used in the field of mental health. A critical examination of the complex relationship between lay and professional ways of describing, assessing and explaining mental distress has revealed how stigmatizing processes dominate both professional discourse and practice and popular culture, and clearly have a negative impact on the lives of the mentally distressed. The over-reliance on the medical model of mental health in contemporary mental health practice has been exposed as heavily problematic and a case has been presented for the more widespread use of the social model of mental health – a model that is more closely aligned to the core values and principles of social work.

Further reading/resources

Foster, J.L.H. (2007) *Journeys Through Mental Illness: Clients' Experiences and Understandings of Mental Distress*. Basingstoke: Palgrave Macmillan.

Laurence, J. (2003) *Pure Madness: How Fear Drives the Mental Health System*. London: Routledge.

Tew, J. (ed.) (2005) *Social Perspectives in Mental Health*. London: Jessica Kingsley Publishers.

www.critpsynet.freeuk.com – the Critical Psychiatry Network.

www.spn.org.uk – the Social Perspectives Network for Modern Mental Health.

www.time-to-change.org.uk – national campaign to end mental health discrimination.

2

THINKING THE PRESENT HISTORICALLY

The making of the modern mental health system

This chapter can be used to support the development of knowledge in professional social work as follows:

National Occupational Standards for Social Work

Key Role 1: Prepare for and work with individuals, families, carers, groups and communities to assess their needs and circumstances

- Prepare for social work contact and involvement.

Key Role 6: Demonstrate professional competence in social work practice

- Research, analyse, evaluate, and use current knowledge of best social work practice.

(TOPSS England, 2002)

Academic Standards for Social Work

Honours graduates in social work:

5.1 should acquire, critically evaluate, apply and integrate knowledge and understanding in relation to:

5.1.1 Social work services, service users and carers

- the social processes (associated with, for example, poverty, migration, unemployment, poor health, disablement, lack of education and other sources of disadvantage) that lead to marginalisation, isolation and exclusion and their impact on the demand for social work services

- explanations of the links between definitional processes contributing to social differences (for example, social class, gender, ethnic differences, age, sexuality and religious belief) to the problems of inequality and differential need faced by service users

- the nature and validity of different definitions of, and explanations for, the characteristics and circumstances of service users and the services required by them, drawing on knowledge from research, practice experience, and from service users and carers.

5.1.2. The service delivery context

- the location of contemporary social work within historical, comparative and global perspectives, including European and international contexts
- the complex relationships between public, social and political philosophies, policies and priorities and the organisation and practice of social work, including the contested nature of these.

5.1.3. Values and ethics

- the nature, historical evolution and application of social work values.

(QAA, 2008)

Key themes in this chapter

- The pre-history of psychiatry
- The beginnings of institutional mental health care
- The madhouse system
- The rise and fall of the asylum
- The establishment of mental hospitals
- The development of social work practice with the mentally distressed
- The transition toward community mental health care.

INTRODUCTION

It is impossible to fully understand the contemporary context of professional practice with the mentally distressed without reference to the origins of the mental health system. With this in mind this chapter aims to trace the historical foundations of service provision, including: the pre-history of psychiatry; the beginnings of state intervention; the madhouse system; the rise and fall of the asylum; the establishment of mental hospitals; the development of social work involvement; and the transition towards community care practice.

From the outset it is important that we acknowledge the plethora of varying and conflicting histories of psychiatry and its development. According to Newnes:

> the way we tell the histories of psychiatric events, practices and ideas changes over time. The comforting accounts of scientific and medical progress, told predominantly by members of the mental health professions themselves, have gradually been replaced by more searching accounts from historians and sociologists. (1999: 20)

Moreover, Porter comments that 'the history of madness is the history of power' (1987a: 39). From early days society has had to draw a balance between care and control for the mentally distressed. Social work is situated between these opposites. As Horner argues 'social work is situated between the powers of statutory intervention and enforcement, and the historic struggles of an oppressed group' (2003: 59).

THE PRE-HISTORY OF PSYCHIATRY

In medieval England there was no systematic approach to the management of the insane. This is perhaps unsurprising given that at this time 'there was no clear definition of what mental disorder was and certainly no recognition of the mentally ill or handicapped as a category requiring a distinct form of treatment' (Jones, 1972: 3).

Case example

Dr William Perfect, who ran a small rest home in Kent, recalled being summoned in 1776 by the parish officers of Friendsbury to see 'a maniacal man they had confined in their workhouse ... He was secured to the floor by means of a staple and an iron ring, which was fastened to a pair of fetters about his legs, and he was handcuffed. Through the bars of his windows continual visitors were pointing at, ridiculing and irritating the patient, who was thus made a spectacle of public sport'.

(taken from Shorter, 1997: 3)

Elizabethan explanations for lunacy were often contradictory – either situated in religious or supernatural beliefs (possession by the devil or divine retribution) or the idea that 'body humours' were imbalanced. It was believed that four basic qualities, namely coldness, dryness, hotness and wetness (represented by the spleen, blood, choler and phlegm) needed to be in balance; imbalance meant disease (Skultans, 1979). The resultant 'treatments' such as blood letting, purges and ceremonies reflect this. Clerics, astrologers, village wizards, folk magicians, and cunning men and women were as likely as surgeons and apothecaries to be summoned to combat the malignity of mental disorder (Scull, 1993).

Many sufferers were left to their own devices. Scull notes 'the beggar wandering from place to place, community to community in search of alms' (1979: 18). Those who presented as too violent or unmanageable for the community were contained in local gaols. Scull further comments that 'efforts were made to keep lunatics, along with the incurably ill, the blind, and the crippled in the community, if necessary by providing their relatives or others who were prepared to care for them with permanent pensions for their support' (1979: 22). Bartlett and Wright point out that the opening paragraph to Scull's *Museums of Madness* demonstrates the 'stark juxtaposition between this open and tolerant care of the insane in pre-industrial communities with that of the restrictive incarceration of the Victorian period' (1999: 1).

> **Group reflection exercise**
>
> Discuss possible reasons why early communities believed that mental illness originated from the devil.

THE BEGINNINGS OF INSTITUTIONAL CARE

There is a general consensus amongst historians of psychiatry that during the first half of the eighteenth century the majority of the insane were to be found in the community as there was as yet no formal segregation of the mad in England. The minority who were confined were either confined under the Poor Laws, vagrancy laws, criminal law, in private madhouses, in Bethlem Hospital (in use since 1377 for those with acute mental disorder financed by public subscription and legacies) or confined alone at their own home. This last category (single lunatics):

> can be divided into three main classes – patients of some social standing who remained in their own home and received medical attention, patients who were 'put away' by their families ... and the family scandal allowed to die down; and those in poorer families who were simply tied or chained in a corner of the house to prevent them becoming a nuisance to other people. The whole object of such confinement was secrecy. (Jones, 1955: 10–11)

Bethlem Royal Hospital (later corrupted to Bedlam) is widely acknowledged to be the first dedicated institution to care for the insane from London and its surrounding areas. From its monastic origins, and being one of the oldest psychiatric hospitals in Europe, it survives today over 750 years later in the form of the Maudsley Hospital which was granted NHS status in 1994. Early images of patients confined in a zoo-like situation, where the London populace visited for entertainment, are forever stuck in the British psyche (Russell, 1997). This reflected another aspect of understanding mental distress in the eighteenth and early nineteenth centuries, which was to compare the mad to animals – violent, insensitive to heat and cold, and lacking in reason.

Case example

Dr William Black (1811) described some of the Bedlam patients as 'ravenous and insatiable as wolves' or 'drenched by compulsion as horses', and the Incurables 'kept as wild beasts, constantly in fetters'. The Parliamentary Commissioners (1815) commented on a room in Bethlem that was like a dog kennel. *The Quarterly Review* (1857) referred to Bethlem patients being enclosed with iron bars, like 'the fiercer carnivore at the Zoological Gardens'.

(taken from Russell, 1997: 5)

Notwithstanding occasional hints of scandal, Bethlem had been a favourite London charity. While there were a few patients from wealthy backgrounds, most were paupers (Scull, 1993). Despite the early scenes of patients suffering brutality, with the regime focusing on control rather than care, pioneering changes were made over the centuries that followed. Yet for all the 'improvements' Russell argues that 'many of the old problems were constantly being recycled – how to manage violence, expressions of sexuality, gender issues, struggles for power between staff and staff, staff and patients, the use of medication, and relationships between the institution and the community' (1997: 213).

THE MADHOUSE SYSTEM

Madhouses were run privately and run for profit, often owned and managed by lay rather than medical proprietors, with a resultant 'trade in lunacy' occurring (Parry-Jones, 1972). They catered for a predominately middle- and upper-class clientele and are known to have existed before the eighteenth century (MacKenzie, 1992). They varied in size from those taking two or three patients to those which accommodated three or four hundred, with the quality of provision ranging from dire to innovative (Jones, 1955). Residents consisted not only of the mad, but also those wrongfully held at the behest of their relatives, as, for example, in the case of women who bore illegitimate children or those who were deemed to be socially embarrassing. As Bartlett and Wright explain, the 'working class and their wealthy counterparts were anxious to conceal the shame of insanity, lest the entire household be stigmatized as insane' (1999: 172). For some the inability to afford madhouse fees and the anxiety about their insane relative becoming public knowledge often resulted in the barbaric containment of the insane in attics and outhouses.

Rogers and Pilgrim note that 'there were sixteen metropolitan licensed houses in 1774 rising rapidly after 1780 but by 1819 there were just forty' (1996: 41). The Metropolitan Commissioners Report of 1844 recorded 37 licensed madhouses in the metropolitan area and on their tour of inspection their chief impression was not one of widespread cruelty and neglect, but of a common evasion of the law. The law relating to the registration of certified persons was often bypassed by proprietors declaring that the patient was merely suffering from 'nerves' (Jones, 1955). Doctors keeping madhouses gained increasing power in managing the insane, with Porter arguing that 'mad doctors all over Europe started to believe that they held madness in their power ... as it was amongst the more curable maladies' (1987a: 41). Commanding, even manhandling, the mad often formed part of the treatment. By 1845 the medical profession had secured powerful support for the proposition that insanity was a disease, and thus was naturally something which doctors alone were qualified to treat (Scull, 1979, 1981).

Despite the conclusions of the 1844 Commissioners Report, some cruelty did exist (Scull, 1996). It was following the suspicious death of a patient called Hannah Mills at the York Asylum in 1791 that the Quaker William Tuke, a wealthy tea and coffee merchant, established a quite different but still privately funded, not for profit, establishment for the care of the mentally ill in 1792. Named neither a hospital nor an asylum, the York Retreat was to be a home where the patient was to be known and treated as an individual and where his/her mind was to be constantly stimulated and encouraged to return to its natural state. Here even the rage of madness could be reigned in without whips, chains, or corporal punishment amidst the comforts of domesticity (Scull, 1996).

Meanwhile in France, Philippe Pinel (considered the founder of modern psychiatry) was also removing chains from patients. Though he had never heard of Tuke, Pinel had also come to the similar conclusion that the key to using the asylum therapeutically lay in 'moral therapy'. Both were instrumental in pioneering more humane ways of treating the mad, supported by the notion that proper care of lunatics was akin to good child care (Porter, 1987a).

THE RISE AND FALL OF THE ASYLUMS

Private, profit-based provision for the mad continued until the coming of the asylums, and only waned when licences were restricted from 1890. In the early part of the nineteenth century reformers such as Lord Shaftesbury, the Tukes, evangelists and philanthropists called for new approaches to the treatment of the insane and fixed on publicly financed asylums, with vigorous inspection by outsiders, as the way forward. The reformers achieved their objectives, but not without 'three decades of Parliamentary manoeuvring, a mass of periodicals and reviews extolling the merits of their proposed solution' (Brown, 1985: 31).

The passing of the County Asylums Act in 1808 enabled public asylums to be financed and built at the discretion of local magistrates. The number of such institutions expanded greatly when the 1845 Lunacy Act made the provision of public asylums compulsory. Asylums soon achieved gigantic proportions, some with facades that stretched for nearly a third of a mile containing wards and passages of more than six miles (Brown, 1985). It was official policy to site asylums in the countryside or in 'retiring' places near towns where land was more readily available, cheaper, and allowed for extensive grounds with plenty of fresh air (Donnelly, 1983). Porter maintains that, 'by the beginning of Victoria's reign psychiatric doctors were even representing the asylum as, potentially at least, more rational, harmonious, and civilized than society itself' (1987a: 156).

By 1890 there were 66 county and borough asylums in England and Wales, each with an average of 802 inmates. In total there were 86,067 officially certified cases of insanity, more than four times as many as 45 years earlier. By 1930 there were nearly 120,000 patients in public asylums and by 1954 there were over 148,000 (Gibbons, 1988). Scull argues, 'the relationship between the construction of asylums and the increase in insanity again suggests that on the whole it was the existence and expansion of the asylum system which created the increased demand for its own services' (1979: 245). Similarly, Porter comments, 'no sooner were asylums built than they were filled to overflowing' (1987a: 20). Torrey (2003) describes this steady increase in the numbers of people identified with a mental illness as 'the invisible plague'.

Each asylum was under the direction of a medical superintendent answerable only to the visiting committee and the Lunacy Commission. Doctors were the officers and nurse attendants were under the control of a matron; a command structure that would last until the 1959 Mental Health Act. While the external architecture of each asylum was often grandiose complete with its own church or chapel, the internal structures were indicative of the then current theory of mental illness (Jones, 1972). The architecture, with its elaborate therapeutic, sanitary and panoptic rationalities was based upon nineteenth-century science as pioneered by William Stark and Andrew Duncan, with Jeremy Bentham and his Panoptican as its patron saint (Porter, 1987a). Donnelly explains:

> the exercise of 'the power of mind over mind' which moral treatment represented to the lunacy reformers depended equally upon the skills of architects; it was their task to prepare the physical spaces of confinement, where in turn physicians could create the proper therapeutic environment' (1983: 48).

Long corridors, large square wards and stout lockable doors made for easy surveillance. Safe seclusion rooms (padded cells) existed and straightjackets were used for the restraint of the most uncontrollable individuals before sedative drugs came to dominate (Scull, 1993). Patients worked on the farms and gardens, in the laundries and sewing rooms; but their work was organized for the maintenance of the institution rather than for their own benefit. They moved from place to place in groups and they were counted in and counted out by nurses who often could not remember names or faces.

Case example

Life … was governed by a rigid regime of sleep, work, eat. Whitewashed walls; plain brick, stone or wooden floors; deal benches and tables; and two WCs for thirty or forty patients provided a fairly cheerless though roomy environment. Windows were generally barred and many wards were locked, although the better asylums gave considerable internal freedom to the inmates.

(taken from Murphy, 1991: 38).

Out of sight and out of mind, such large numbers were incarcerated in this way in England and across Europe that Foucault describes this as 'the great confinement'. Madness was thus 'left' at the asylum with 'confinement seen as its natural abode' (1967: 36).

Initial enlightened ideas and the promise of cures turned sour. Shorter argues that 'the rise of the asylums is the story of good intentions gone bad' (1997: 33). By the start of the First World War asylums had become vast warehouses for the chronically insane and demented. Controversy exists about the reasons for this failure, with some arguing that the sheer weight of numbers was the problem, caused by two components – a genuine increase in psychiatric illness, and a 'redistribution effect' where individuals were shifted from the family and the workhouse to the asylum (Bynum et al., 1985; Shorter, 1997). Others argue that the increase was due to capitalist society avenging itself on the patients for their unwillingness to work. Society's growing intolerance of deviance thus led to greater confinement of intolerable individuals (Szasz, 1961).

The 1890 Lunacy Act formalized the process of admission to asylums in order to safeguard against illegal detainment. However, Jones maintains that 'from a medical point of view it was out of date before it was passed' (1972: 226). A situation of legalism versus custodialism had occurred. Because of concerns about civil rights, asylums could only take certified patients, who could only be certified when it was obvious to a justice of the peace that they needed containment. By this point, the principles of early diagnosis and the treatment of mild or acute cases had been lost; the asylum's work thus became largely custodial. Rogers and Pilgrim argue that, in the wake of this Act, 'psychiatry settled down as a paternalistic asylum based discipline with little to show for itself as a medical specialism offering genuine cures for madness' (1996: 51).

Reflection exercise

Why would the Victorians believe that institutional care was the best provision for the mentally distressed? Why did this view change?

THE ESTABLISHMENT OF MENTAL HOSPITALS

The start of the twentieth century was to witness further controversy concerning the treatment of the mentally distressed, not least from the effects of the First World War (1914–18). As a result of the experiences of war, many soldiers were suffering breakdown (shellshock), with figures showing that this was more prevalent among upper-middle-class officers (Rogers and Pilgrim, 1996). This caused a crisis for the existing services that had until this point been based on bio-deterministic ideas and institutional containment. Government and psychiatrists were forced to turn their attention to stress conditions that were self-evidently environmental, the victims of which were deemed to be 'honourable' and not 'degenerate'.

After the First World War 'conditions in the mental hospitals, as they were now being increasingly called, began to improve again' (Jones, 1993: 126). Though the 1890 Lunacy Act was still in force, its Commission was replaced under the 1913 Mental Deficiency Act by the Board of Control which was to deal with both mental illness and mental deficiency. Responsibility for the oversight of the Board was transferred from the Lord Chancellor's Department to the Home Office; a move that Jones argues 'was away from legal control' (1993: 124). In 1919 the Ministry of Health was set up; the same year the Board of Control drafted a Report for the government Reconstruction Committee which made major recommendations for the future. These included: treatment in mental hospitals without certification; establishing psychiatric units and out-patient clinics in general hospitals; and the provision of funds to voluntary societies for aftercare (Jones, 1993). These recommendations and public discussion about the 1922 Prestwich Hospital Inquiry into allegations of poor treatment, led to the establishment of a Royal Commission in 1924 chaired by Hugh Pattison (later

Lord Macmillan). The Macmillan Commission was to inquire into certification and detention of people who were of unsound mind, and into treatment without certification for people with a mental disorder.

The Commission reported in 1926 and re-stated the principles stated earlier by the Board of Control. Though the Commission was critical of aspects of the system it rejected suggestions that there were widespread infringements of liberty. They recommended voluntary admission on the written application of the patient without medical recommendation, but once admitted, discharge would be subject to a requirement of 72 hours notice. They also proposed greater protection for doctors against accusations of acting in bad faith or without reasonable care (Fennell, 1996). Rogers and Pilgrim argue that the Commission's position was one:

> which is still bedevilling modern attempts to make therapeutic law. On the one hand there was an emphasis on the need for benign care, curative intent and consideration for the sufferers' needs. On the other hand, the emphasis on the need for the use of force in the case of mental illness actually requires the deprivation of liberty without trial: the removal of a fundamental civil right. (1996: 55)

The 1930 Mental Treatment Act that followed the Macmillan Commission incorporated such contradiction. While certification procedures continued under the 1890 Act, two new categories of patient admission were introduced. A 'voluntary patient' could make a written application for treatment and discharge themselves with 72 hours notice. 'Temporary patients' were defined as persons 'suffering from mental illness and likely to benefit by temporary treatment, but for the time being incapable of expressing (themselves) as willing or unwilling to receive such treatment' (Jones, 1993: 135). Psychiatric out-patient clinics were to be funded and new terminology was to be used. The asylum name was to be replaced by 'mental hospital' or simple 'hospital' and the term 'lunatic' by 'person of unsound mind'. The Macmillan reforms went ahead with voluntary admissions reaching 35.2 per cent of all admissions by 1938 and out-patient clinics attached to general hospitals increasing in number. Staffing numbers improved and there were moves to have more unlocked wards except for very disturbed patients (Jones, 1993). Systems of parole were used for patients and professional training improved along with 'social workers' carrying out domiciliary visits.

THE DEVELOPMENT OF SOCIAL WORK PRACTICE WITH THE MENTALLY DISTRESSED

Britain was among the first societies to have identifiable social work activity. It originally manifested itself in the final quarter of the nineteenth century as voluntary (and predominantly female) work and it focused on the undesirable consequences of industrialization and urbanization (Jordan, 1997). Social problems such as ill health and disease, poor housing, overcrowding, prostitution, abuse of children and alcohol abuse, which were largely invisible in the countryside, became commonplace in the towns and cities. Living conditions for the poor in major towns and cities were squalid, unsanitary, poorly ventilated and dangerous to health. Poverty was rife and the absence of available work often meant the difference between living and literally starving. Frederick Engels visited England from 1842 to 1844 and described his observations in graphic detail – 'in every manufacturing town there is to be seen, a multitude of people, especially women and children going about barefoot' (1973: 97). Life was short for both children and adults. In Manchester, for example, 'more than fifty seven per cent of the children of the working class perish before their fifth year' (1973: 131). For adults, official figures for 1839–40 show that for every 45 members of the population, one died every year (Engels, 1973).

Middle-class city dwellers perceived dangers from the social deprivation experienced by the working classes and called for something to be done to contain and control this threat from the 'dangerous classes'. The response was a variety of state social welfare initiatives which were created in the nineteenth century. Public schemes for sanitation, education, prisons, policing, workhouses and asylums for the mentally ill were all created. Despite many families only surviving with the support of charity, concern focused yet again on the 'deserving' and the 'undeserving poor'. In 1870 the London Charity Organisation Society was established to both provide principles for, and to coordinate, charitable giving and to repress mendicity (idleness). Assessment and help were based around a family's 'character', with past histories and records being kept. Viewed by many as the beginning of 'social work' in society, Payne argues that 'this was the beginning of ... assessment as a bedrock of social work practice' (2005: 36).

Psychiatric social work (PSW) developed as a practice mainly in mental hospitals and child guidance clinics between the wars around the 1930s. The Tavistock Clinic founded in 1920 also used social workers, initially to support and assist the recovery of shellshocked patients, but moved on to provide specialist analytical training and support for mental health workers. As welfare activities expanded during the inter-war years elements of social work were drawn into the operations of the state. Probation was tied up with the legal system; almoners were operating on the margins of the nursing and medical professions, while mental health workers were in a field of practice dominated by the psychiatric profession (Clarke, 1993).

As with the First World War, the Second World War brought great upheaval and new psychiatric problems. Again, men working in the mental health system (doctors, nurses, porters) were enrolled to assist in the war effort. Jones (1993) notes that over half of the accommodation in mental hospitals was taken over for emergency purposes, out-patient clinics collapsed for want of staff and, though it did not happen, there was considerable apprehension that there may be mass panic and widespread mental breakdown. Before the war was over, William Beveridge's *Report on Social Insurance and Allied Services* was published (1942), directed at the abolition of squalor, want, ignorance, disease and idleness. The new proposals had three central themes, namely, full employment, the provision of children's allowances and the establishment of a National Health Service which would be 'free at the point of delivery', all paid for by a National Insurance Scheme. At first it was not decided whether mental hospitals were to be incorporated into the NHS scheme but the 1944 White Paper *A National Health Service* and a joint Psychological Association and Royal College of Physicians Report, *The Future Organization of Psychiatric Services*, in 1945, both argued for its inclusion. As a result, Jones argues that 'the artificial divorce between the treatment of the mind and the treatment of the body would be ended, and the gap between the treatment of the psychoses (largely in county mental hospitals) and the treatment of the neuroses (largely in voluntary hospitals and private practice) would be bridged' (1993: 143). Reform of the existing mental health services was called for and the government's response was to set up the Royal Commission on Mental Illness and Mental Deficiency in 1954. The Commission reported in 1957 and the resulting Bill put before the Lords was introduced by Lord Hailsham who described it as 'the first fundamental revision of the English mental health laws since 1845' (Jones, 1993: 156). The Mental Health Act 1959 which followed created a new basis for the treatment of mental distress as an 'illness' essentially akin to any physical illness (Jones, 1993). Rivett comments that 'the Act aimed to break down segregation, and the feelings of isolation, neglect and frustration. Services would now be planned across hospital and community boundaries, by specialists, family doctors, and local authority staff, nurses and social workers' (1997: 159). An awareness of institutionalization led many to believe that it was in the best interests of those who could to live in the community, and local authorities began expanding domiciliary services, hostels, day centres, social clubs and day hospitals for the mentally ill with this objective in mind.

Irvine notes that during the 1950s, 'demand for PSWs had spread far outside the bounds of mental hospitals and child guidance clinics with debate existing about whether they were primarily social workers or therapists' (1978: 176). Either way, their energy and initiative in pioneering community care schemes contributed to the increasing role played by social workers. Although medicine was the primary profession dealing with mental disorder, 'social work increasingly played a complementary role when from the 1950s the profound influence which the family and social environment had on the well being and level of social functioning of mentally disordered people became clearer' (Younghusband, 1978: 165).

The 1957 Royal Commission on the Law relating to Mental Illness and Mental Deficiency thought that social work with the families of in-patients was desirable and that social work for patients not receiving hospital treatment, including those who had left hospital, should be the responsibility of the local authorities. This had the effect of greatly increasing the demand for social workers and trained staff in homes and hostels – a demand that was to continue over the coming decades. Titmuss observes that 'whenever the British people have identified a social problem there has followed a national call for more social work and more trained social workers' (1968: 85). Similarly, Walton states that 'for much of the second half of the twentieth century, social work education and training have been insufficient in quantity and quality to match the increasing demands on the profession' (1975: 209).

The Mental Health Act 1959 established the appointment of social workers as Mental Welfare Officers to carry out duties in relation to the Act. The Act had abolished the distinction between psychiatric and other hospitals and encouraged the development of care in the community. Mental Welfare Officers, employed by local authorities, were to play a key role in achieving this objective, for in addition to arranging compulsory admission when necessary and attending Mental Health Tribunals, they could arrange guardianship for private individuals. They supported individuals in the community by carrying out routine family visits, monitoring progress, arranging day care centre placements and social club attendance, and assisting with employment. In 1961, returns to the Ministry of Health showed that 1,128 mental health social workers were employed by 146 local authorities in England and Wales (Younghusband, 1978). Despite this, many more social workers were needed and there was something of a staff shortage. Younghusband (1978) observes that in 1967 nearly 185,000 mentally ill or retarded people were receiving local authority mental health services, in close cooperation with mental hospitals and GPs. Seventy-one day care centres and 247 social clubs were also in place.

Though many of the large hospitals had closed, others were closing, and many more people were being cared for in the community. Community care was itself still an objective. The Seebohm Report stated:

> the widespread belief that we have 'community care' of the mentally disordered is, for many parts of the country, still a sad illusion [and that] social workers should be concerned with the whole family, learning how to make a family diagnosis, and be able to take wide responsibility and mobilize a wide range of services. (Seebohm, 1968: paras 353 and 339)

Seebohm's recommendations for the establishment of social service departments were implemented in the 1970 Local Authority Social Services Act, but notably 'none of the first round of Directors appointed came from the mental health field' (Jones, 1993: 187). The Act contained the notion of 'generic' social work, but there was much opposition to the reorganization which separated mental health social workers, hostels, day care and other services from the other local authority mental health services. Danbury (1976) gave evidence of the difficulties some social workers faced at the time because they were unfamiliar with the regulations and procedures, were afraid of the patients, and had received no in-service training. As a result of the pressure applied by Seebohm and the newly formed British Association of Social Workers, the Central Council for Education and Training in Social Work (CCETSW) was formed in 1971. That same year CCETSW introduced the Certificate of Qualification in Social Work (CQSW), the first universally recognized professional qualification in social work in Britain. Thus as Langan suggests, 'the modern social worker came into existence as an amalgam of half a dozen or more occupational groups – psychiatric and medical social workers, and "officers" concerned with offenders, children, mental health, housing and educational welfare' (1993: 50).

Reflection exercise

What concerns do you think mental health social workers had about the formation of the 'new' social service departments arising from the 1970 Local Authority Social Services Act?

The 1970s are seen now as the 'glory days' of social work when there was both ideological and legislative support for social work as a profession in its own right, and when numbers of social workers increased from 10,346 in 1971 to 21,182 in 1976 (NALGO, 1989). This was not to last however, and the glory days were soon over with social workers facing a new anti-welfare Conservative government that came to power in 1979, and finding themselves on strike during the latter part of the decade. The Barclay Committee was set up in 1980 to examine the crisis that social work found itself in. It reported in 1982 stating that:

> Too much is expected of social workers. We load upon them unrealistic expectations and then we complain when they do not live up to them. Social work is a relatively young profession. It has grown rapidly as the flow of legislation has greatly increased the range and complexity of its work. (Barclay, 1982: vii)

Langan argues, 'the Barclay Report attempted to reconcile Seebohm and the new right, and inevitably failed' (cited in Clarke, 1993: 63). Furthermore, the two minority reports that accompanied the main report both assumed the demise of the generic social worker as the dominant force in the provision of social support. Nevertheless, in the middle of this period the DHSS White Paper *Better Services for the Mentally Ill* confirmed the importance of the social worker's role in working with the mentally distressed when it stated, 'the unifying element ... is the professional skill of the social worker, whether deployed in fieldwork, in primary care, in residential or day care, or in hospital' (DHSS, 1975: 23).

The Mental Health Act 1959 had governed the process of admission to psychiatric hospital for 24 years, but, as Davies maintains, 'it came under increasing attack partly because of the way the facility for emergency admissions was abused and partly because of the ambiguous role of the social worker in the process' (1981: 114). The Mental Health Act 1983 was designed to improve matters with a statutory requirement for 'approved social workers' (ASWs) to be properly trained, and in order to fulfill their role they would be required to carry out professional assessments. The minimum requirement to become an ASW was two years relevant post-qualifying experience and the completion of a specialist training course. Thus, the specific role assigned to Mental Welfare Officers under the 1959 Act was made clearer for Approved Social Workers under the 1983 Act, albeit with their powers controlled by strict time limits stated in the legislation and supervised by the courts, subject to medical collaboration, and with the rights of patients and their families protected. This nevertheless created an important and specific role for one group of social workers at a time of nervousness in the profession.

THE TRANSITION TO COMMUNITY MENTAL HEALTH CARE

As outlined earlier the major move toward care in the community came with the emptying of the asylums. The number of residents in the asylums peaked at around 150,000 in 1955, but by 1992 this figure had plummeted to just 50,000. Much has been written concerning deinstitutionalization of the mentally ill with various commentators speculating as to the primary motivating force(s) underpinning the process of change (Busfield, 1986; Jones, 1993; Scull, 1977). Four main drivers have been identified, as follows.

The Drug Revolution

It is widely believed that it was the 'scientific breakthrough' in the development of the major tranquillizing drugs in the 1950s that enabled large numbers of mental patients to be discharged into the community. However, many of these drugs were not widely used until some years after patients had already begun to be transferred to the community. Scull (1977) argues that while drug treatments may have facilitated the management of mental patients discharged into the community, they were not responsible for community care policy as such.

Therapeutic Optimism

After the Second World War many psychoanalytically oriented army psychiatrists such as Tom Main, Maxwell Jones and David Clarke led the way in pioneering new approaches to mental distress. 'Therapeutic communities' were developed and the same pioneers set about unlocking the doors of the traditional mental hospitals in an effort to humanize the care and treatment of the institutionalized insane. By the 1950s most hospitals had open door policies.

Anti-institutional Critiques

From the 1950s onwards a growing body of critical work emerged that reflected a profound disenchantment with institutional care in all its forms. Writings on the sociology of deviance, phenomenology, ethnomethodology, labelling theory and symbolic interactionism (for example Goffman, 1961; Laing, 1959; Scheff, 1966; Szasz, 1961) not only represented a powerful critical literature around the nature, causes and responses to mental distress but also contributed to the call for deinstitutionalization.

Economic Crisis

Scull's (1977: 1) preferred explanation for what he refers to as the 'state sponsored policy of closing down asylums' is an economic one. He argues that the social control mechanism of segregation that epitomized the nineteenth-century approach to managing the mad became an increasing financial burden to the state that could not be sustained; therefore propelling patients from segregation in the asylum to neglect in the community. Busfield (1986) suggests that Scull's argument fails to account for increases in expenditure on mental health services during this period – especially in relation to primary care. However, she does acknowledge that this expenditure was skewed towards services for people with less severe mental health problems at the expense of the chronically mentally distressed.

It is likely that deinstitutionalization was, to a greater or lesser extent, a consequence of all of the above. Regardless, the expansion of state medical and social services meant that the institutional setting became less significant and no longer represented the ideal location for psychiatric practice. Yet if the intention was that with the closure of the large institutions patients would find themselves in a new, less institutionalized, more therapeutic environment, the reality was that many of the theories and practices of the asylum transferred with them (Rogers and Pilgrim, 2001). Moreover, by the late 1970s it was clear that the state's interpretation of community care was changing.

In the broader context of fiscal crisis and economic recession a 'New Right' Conservative government had come into power in 1979 with an 'anti-welfarist agenda' high on its list of priorities. The stated objective of Margaret Thatcher's government during the 1980s and early 1990s was to roll back the 'nanny state'. As far as social workers were concerned, Cochrane quotes a senior Minister (John Patten) reported in *The Times* in 1991 as arguing that, 'municipal armies of social workers should be disbanded and responsibility for caring for the vulnerable and inadequate transferred to smaller community-based groups' (1993: 73). Sir Roy Griffiths was given the task of reviewing the efficiency of public organizations, and his Report, *Community Care: An Agenda for Action* was published in 1988. The Report proposed ways of introducing community care linked to reducing levels of public expenditure, and, as Clarke notes, 'the Griffiths Report acknowledges that the new arrangements are likely to change the ways in which professionals – and social workers in particular – will have to operate' (1993:79).

The government's White Paper *Caring for People* followed and incorporated Griffiths' ideas on the purchaser/provider split, encouraging local authorities to construct care packages that should 'make use wherever possible of services from voluntary, "not for profit" and private providers insofar as this represents a cost-effective care choice' (DH, 1989: 22). As Means and Smith (1998) argue, the White Paper was not received favourably and some criticized it as part of a Thatcherite strategy to introduce the market to public services. The NHS and Community Care Act 1990 that followed, 'changed the traditional territory of the mental health professions' (Rogers and Pilgrim, 2001: 89), and brought with it new funding regimes which social workers were required to re-orientate themselves to. The Act heralded a shift away from the post-war pattern of welfare services where the state played the central role, to a 'mixed economy of welfare' in which the voluntary, informal and private sectors would play a greater part. As Clarke maintains, it signalled the 'end to the social services department as a 'monopolistic provider' of services' (1993: 151). Services would be 'needs led' and 'clients' would become 'customers'; social workers would become 'care managers', assessing customers' needs and purchasing services on their behalf from the local mixed economy of care. Means and Smith argue that 'these were under-funded regimes … that had new complex assessment and fee payment systems which depended upon the willingness of social workers and other field-level staff to take an increased role in the means testing of clients' (1998: 107). Social workers became uneasy with their new role as budget managers, with Langan and Means (1995) finding that many social workers resented the 'money role' being passed on to them. The care management approach changed the very nature of social work. The primary objective of achieving a trusting, caring and supportive relationship with clients was replaced with a customer–service provider relationship. That social workers in mental health services put together 'care packages' within a community care framework within set budgets, in what Harris describes as 'the social work business' (2003: 1), is the subject of Chapter 3.

CHAPTER SUMMARY

The development of the modern mental health system has a complex and convoluted history. Accounts of that history are inevitably tainted with the subjective meanings and interpretations of those contributing to it. There are therefore *multiple histories* reflecting the legacy of ideas, institutions and practices of each generation. Given this, the simplicity of the summary of the early development of mental health provision in Britain offered by Kathleen Jones has an obvious appeal: 'In the eighteenth century, madmen were locked up in madhouses: in the nineteenth century, lunatics were sent to asylums; and in the twentieth century, the mentally ill receive treatment in hospitals' (1955: ix). To which may be added that in the late twentieth and early twenty-first centuries the mentally distressed were cared for in the community. Whether the ideal of 'community care' has actually been achieved remains a matter of significant debate and is the subject of the next chapter.

Further reading/resources

Coppock, V. and Hopton, J. (2000) *Critical Perspectives on Mental Health*. London: Routledge.
Porter, R. (2002) *Madness: a Brief History*. Oxford: Oxford University Press.
Rogers, A. and Pilgrim, D. (2001) *Mental Health Policy in Britain*, 2nd edn. Basingstoke: Macmillan

3

CARE IN THE COMMUNITY

Policy ideals and practice realities

This chapter can be used to support the development of knowledge and skills in professional social work as follows:

National Occupational Standards for Social Work

Key Role 1: Prepare for and work with individuals, families, carers, groups and communities to assess their needs and circumstances

- Prepare for social work contact and involvement
- Work with individuals, families, carers, groups and communities to help them make informed decisions
- Assess needs and options to recommend a course of action.

Key Role 2: Plan, carry out, review and evaluate social work practice, with individuals, families, carers, groups and communities and other professionals

- Interact with individuals, families, carers, groups and communities to achieve change and development and to improve life opportunities
- Prepare, produce, implement and evaluate plans with individuals, families, carers, groups, communities and professional colleagues
- Support the development of networks to meet assessed needs and planned outcomes
- Work with groups to promote individual growth, development and independence.

Key Role 3: Support individuals to represent their needs, views and circumstances

- Advocate with, and on behalf of, individuals, families, carers, groups and communities
- Prepare for, and participate in decision making forums.

Key Role 4: Manage risk to individuals, families, carers, groups, communities, self and colleagues

- Assess and manage risks to individuals, families, carers, groups and communities.

Key Role 5: Manage and be accountable, with supervision and support, for your own social work practice within your organisation

- Work within multi-disciplinary and multi-organisational teams, networks and systems.

(TOPPS England, 2002)

Academic Standards for Social Work

Honours graduates in social work:

4.6 must learn to:

- recognise and work with the powerful links between intrapersonal and interpersonal factors and the wider social, legal, economic, political and cultural context of people's lives.

4.7 should learn to become accountable, reflective, critical and evaluative which involves learning to:

- work in a transparent and responsible way, balancing autonomy with complex, multiple and sometimes contradictory accountabilities (for example, to different service users, employing agencies, professional bodies and the wider society).

5.1 should acquire, critically evaluate, apply and integrate knowledge and understanding in relation to:

5.1.2 The service delivery context

- the complex relationships between public, social and political philosophies, policies and priorities and the organisation and practice of social work, including the contested nature of these
- the issues and trends in modern public and social policy and their relationship to contemporary practice and service delivery in social work
- the current range and appropriateness of statutory, voluntary and private agencies providing community-based, day-care, residential and other services and the organisational systems inherent within these
- the significance of interrelationships with other social services, especially education, housing, health, income maintenance and criminal justice.

5.1.3 Values and ethics

- the complex relationships between justice, care and control in social welfare and the practical and ethical implications of these, including roles as statutory agents and in upholding the law in respect of discrimination.

5.1.4 Social work theory

- models and methods of assessment, including factors underpinning the selection and testing of relevant information, the nature of professional judgement and the processes of risk assessment and decision-making
- approaches and methods of intervention in a range of settings, including factors guiding the choice and evaluation of these.

5.1.5 The nature of social work practice

- the characteristics of practice in a range of community-based and organisational settings including group-care, within statutory, voluntary and private sectors, and the factors influencing changes and developments in practice within these contexts.

(QAA, 2008)

Key themes in this chapter

- What is meant by 'community care'?
- Who provides community care?
- Community care policy and legislation in the 1990s
- 'Scare' in the community – the media, moral panics and community care
- New Labour's modernization of mental health services
- Community Mental Health Teams and the modern Care Programme Approach
- The 'Personalization Agenda' and mental health care

INTRODUCTION

In Chapter 2 we established the 'long history' of the mental health system in the UK concluding with the origins and background to the provision of community care for the mentally distressed. In this chapter we trace the implementation and further development of community care policy and practice for the mentally distressed from the early 1990s to the present. We begin by highlighting the ambiguities that lay behind the terms 'community' and 'care', as well as the concept of 'community care' itself, acknowledging the role of informal care that is provided by relatives, friends, neighbours and volunteers. Building on the discussion from the latter part of Chapter 2 we move on to critically evaluate the implementation of the NHS and Community Care Act 1990 with particular emphasis on the complex and contradictory relationship between the care management role of local authority social services departments and the NHS-led Care Progamme Approach. The confusion around 'who does what?' in providing community care for the mentally distressed contributed in no small part to the high profile tragedies of the 1990s. The role of the media in cultivating a climate of fear amongst the general public around community care for the mentally distressed is also explored. The chapter moves on to outline the 'modernization' policy reforms introduced by the New Labour government from the late 1990s onwards, including the *National Service Framework for Mental Health* (*NSFMH*) (DH, 1999a) and the modern Care Programme Approach (CPA). The chapter concludes with a critical discussion around New Labour's 'personalization agenda' as it relates to those in mental distress.

WHAT IS MEANT BY 'COMMUNITY CARE'?

Though the NHS and Community Care Act 1990 has the words 'community' and 'care' in its title, there has always been debate about what these individual words, as well as the phrase itself, actually mean. As Sharkey simply states, 'community care is hard to define' (2007: 1).

> **Reflection exercise**
>
> What does the word 'care' mean to you? What does the word 'community' mean to you? How would you define 'community care'?

In 1978, Jones, Brown and Bradshaw gave a challenging definition of community care:

> To the politician community care is a useful piece of rhetoric. To the sociologist it is a stick to beat institutional care with; to the civil servant it is a cheap alternative to institutional care which can be passed on to the local authorities for action, or inaction. To the visionary it is a dream of a new society in which people do care; to social services departments it is a nightmare of heightened public expectations and inadequate resources to meet them. We are only just beginning to find out what it means to the old, the chronically sick and the handicapped. (1978: 114)

In many respects it could be argued that the same tensions in understanding community care apply as much now as then, some 30 years later.

WHO PROVIDES COMMUNITY CARE?

When thinking about and using the term 'community care' distinctions also need to be made between care *in* and care *by* the community. Care *in* the community usually refers to the various sources of care provided by local authorities, the NHS, private and voluntary organizations – primarily under the provisions of the NHS and Community Care Act 1990 (and in relation to mental health, under the aftercare provisions of the Mental Health Act 1983). Care *by* the community is often taken to mean the informal care provided by community members themselves such as family, friends, neighbours and volunteers. In reality, the majority of community care is provided by these people. The 2001 Census indicated that there are some 6 million carers in the UK and, according to Glendinning and Arksey (2008), the care they provide is worth an estimated £87 billion. The mental health charity Rethink estimates that there are 1.5 million mental health carers (Rethink, 2003).

> ### Reflection exercise: the impact of mental distress and caring
>
> Imagine a person very close to you is given a diagnosis of schizophrenia.
>
> How do you think your life would change? What new or different caring tasks might you need to take on? What resources and services do you think you would need to support you in caring?

It is only relatively recently that the role of carers has been formally acknowledged in government policy and legislation. This is in no small part due to the contribution of feminist researchers who, during the 1980s, revealed the hidden army of carers propping up the welfare state. Significantly, they also revealed that the majority of care was provided by women (Finch and Groves, 1983; Ungerson, 1987). The 2001 Census shows that 58 per cent of carers are women.

> ### Key policy and legislation relating to carers
>
> 1989 Caring for People: Community Care in the Next Decade and Beyond
> 1995 The Carers (Recognition and Services) Act
> 1998 National Carers Strategy
> 1999 National Service Framework for Mental Health (Standard 6)
> 2000 Carers and Disabled Children Act
> 2004 Carers (Equal Opportunities) Act
> 2008 Carers at the Heart of 21st Century Families and Communities: a Caring System on Your Side, a Life of Your Own (the revised National Carers Strategy)

The Carers (Recognition and Services) Act came into force April 1996. For the first time this Act stipulated that those providing 'regular and substantial care' were entitled to request an assessment of their ability to care (a carer's assessment). The New Labour government introduced a National Carers Strategy in 1998 with the aim of improving information, support and care for all carers and the National Service Framework for Mental Health (NSFMH) (DH, 1999a) included a specific standard relating to carers. Standard 6 states that all individuals who provide regular and substantial care for a person on the Care Programme Approach (CPA) should have an assessment of their caring, physical and mental health needs repeated on at least an annual basis and have their own written care plan which is given to them and implemented in discussion with them. The entitlement to an assessment (and to be informed of that right) was strengthened by the Carers and Disabled Children Act 2000 and the Carers (Equal Opportunities) Act 2004. The latter also required local authorities take account of carers' outside interests and that NHS and social services work together more effectively to provide support to carers. While these positive developments have been welcomed by carers, their implementation has often fallen short of expectations. Research has demonstrated that those who care for the mentally distressed are particularly vulnerable and their needs frequently overlooked (Aldridge and Becker, 2003; Arksey et al., 2002; Hogman and Pearson, 1995; Perring et al., 1990; Rethink, 2003; Singleton et al., 2002). A revised National Carers Strategy was introduced in June 2008 which outlines a set of commitments and a 10-year vision of what support for carers should be like by 2018 (DH, 2008a).

The revised National Carers Strategy 2008

By 2018:

- carers will be respected as expert care partners and will have access to the integrated and personalized services they need to support them in their caring role
- carers will be able to have a life of their own alongside their caring role
- carers will be supported so that they are not forced into financial hardship by their caring role
- carers will be supported to stay mentally and physically well and treated with dignity
- children and young people will be protected from inappropriate caring and have the support they need to learn, develop and thrive, to enjoy positive childhoods and to achieve against all the Every Child Matters outcomes.

COMMUNITY CARE FOR THE MENTALLY DISTRESSED IN THE 1990S

Key policy relating to community care for the mentally distressed 1986–1996

1986 Making a Reality of Community Care
1988 Community Care: An Agenda for Action (The Griffiths Report)
1989 Caring for People: Community Care in the Next Decade and Beyond
1990 NHS and Community Care Act
1991 Care Programme Approach (CPA) introduced
1994 Supervision Registers introduced
1994 Guidance on the Discharge of Mentally Disordered People and their Continuing Care in the Community
1995 Disability Discrimination Act
1995 Mental Health (Patients in the Community) Act 1995
1996 The Community Care (Direct Payments) Act

As we established in Chapter 2, the NHS and Community Care Act 1990 brought unprecedented structural changes to the delivery of health and social care services in the UK. Driven essentially by an ideological commitment to reducing the role of the state in the provision of services and a belief that the market is the most efficient way of matching resources to need, the Act introduced a business-oriented approach via mechanisms such as: compulsory competitive tendering; the creation of the purchaser-provider split; the introduction of GP fund-holding and self-governing hospital trusts; and a drive towards quantitative measures of services and outputs in what has been termed the 'commodification' of welfare (Le Grand, 1993; Offe, 1984). Those formerly called 'patients' now became 'service users', reflecting the ideological shift not only in the relationship between the state and its citizens but also between health and social care professionals and their clients.

The quasi-market system introduced in the UK operates through 'care managers'. The 'case management' approach was imported into Britain from the USA and Canada. The approach was piloted during the 1970s and 1980s by the University of Kent's Personal Social Services Research Unit with the aim of showing how case managers holding their own budgets could provide better tailored services and support. The practice involves a single worker (not necessarily a social worker) assessing, coordinating and purchasing care for a client. Here the worker acts as a kind of 'broker' aiming to achieve the best deal for their client, as with purchasing insurance or travel. It also involves budgets and budget management which in many ways is seen as alien to the role of a social worker. The policy guidance to the NHS and Community Care Act 1990 set out the role of care management:

- to ensure that available resources are used effectively
- to restore and maintain independence by enabling people to live in the community
- to minimize the effects of disability and illness
- to treat service users respectfully and provide equal opportunities
- to promote individual choice and self determination, and build on existing strengths and care resources
- to promote partnership between users, carers, and service providers and the organizations representing them.

Central to the implementation of care management is the assessment of 'need'. However, as Payne points out, it is need that is defined by the care agency or authority and not by the service user, and the definition of need is set within the context of control of expenditure (cited in Bornat et al., 1997). Harris takes this further and argues that social work has been made a business, with 'community care being used as the primary vehicle for this to occur through the inter-related developments of marketisation and managerialism' (2003: 33). Dustin (2007) refers to this process as the 'McDonaldisation' of social work. Such changes shifted the locus of power from professional to managerial control – functions that were previously the domain of finance and administration sections in local authority social services departments.

Somewhat ironically, the introduction of needs-led provision was in part a response to the criticism that the provision of services had traditionally been dominated by professionals and was not properly organized to meet the needs of service users who, after all, were in the best position to identify their own needs. The intention was to move away from 'this is what we offer' towards local authorities asking 'what do you need? As time would prove, however, this did not mean that users would always get what they wanted or needed. Needs-led assessments raised the expectations and hopes of users which then had to be tempered by the harsh realities of budget constraints and long waiting lists. Local authority managers soon became preoccupied with the management of scarce resources as they attempted to balance competing demands and tried to make ends meet. Lewis and Glennerster point out that many social workers were initially enthusiastic that a needs-led service would result in user empowerment, but those same workers 'have found it difficult to separate needs led based assessment from the ever present issue of resources and what services are actually available' (1998: 206).

Community care for people in mental distress is not only based on the premise that needs-led assessments will lead to the provision of 'appropriate' services, for needs-led assessments to work there has to be effective cooperation between the various agencies involved. While the rhetoric of government ministers in the 1990s focused on a commitment to giving people who use mental health services more of a say, the reality highlighted a system plagued by gross under-funding and role confusion. The NHS-led Care Programme Approach (CPA), introduced in 1991 (the same time as local authorities were implementing care management under the NHS and Community Care Act 1990), was also intended to provide a framework for the care of those in mental distress outside hospital, in the community. All patients seen by specialist mental health services were to have their need for treatment assessed, a care plan drawn up and a named 'key' mental health worker to coordinate their care, including a regular review of their needs. The Care Programme Approach was intended to provide continuity of care for the mentally distressed across different services and so required health and local authorities to work together. However, as Hannigan states:

> Confusingly, both care management and CPA were introduced as mechanisms through which multi-disciplinary and multi-agency continuity of care could be organised and delivered. In many areas the lack of integration between the two methods resulted in duplication of effort, excessive bureaucracy and construction of a barrier to effective joint working. (2003: 32)

Although social services were designated as the lead agency for the community care of people with mental health problems and health authorities would remain responsible for the 'health' element of care, the meaning of 'lead agency' and the distinction between social care and health care was never clarified. Inevitably, the conflicts that followed around who should be responsible for what affected the quality of care received by those in mental distress. As Muijen observes, 'mental health care was indeed – as Sir Roy Griffiths had predicted – "everybody's distant relative but nobody's baby"' (1995: 41). Evaluative research post-implementation reinforced the suspicion that the system was not working and the mentally distressed were being alienated rather than integrated in the community (Repper et al., 1997; Taylor, 1994/95).

'SCARE' IN THE COMMUNITY: THE MEDIA AND MORAL PANICS AROUND COMMUNITY CARE

By early 1994 the debate around community care rapidly became entangled in a series of moral panics surrounding a small number of high profile tragedies, including those of Ben Silcock, Michael Buchanan and Christopher Clunis. The long-standing ethical and moral dilemma of protection of the public versus preserving the civil and human rights of the mentally distressed was brought sharply back into focus. Fuelled by media frenzy, with headlines such as 'Freed to Kill in the Community' (*Daily Mail*, 2 July 1993), the impression was created of there being widespread danger from mental patients in the community and particularly from black patients: 'Readers and television viewers are left with subconscious associations between the spectre of unprovoked, inexplicable murder in the street and black psychiatric patients, a potentially explosive combination' (Francis, 1996: 4). Inevitably the debate shifted away from the potential benefits of community care for the mentally distressed and moved towards the issues of 'risk' and 'dangerousness' with calls for greater controls – both for the protection of the public and for the protection of the mentally distressed themselves (Pilgrim and Rogers, 1996). This shift in focus and the ensuing problems surrounding the assessment of 'risk' and 'dangerousness' in mental health practice will be discussed in the wider context of mental health law in Chapter 4.

As has frequently occurred in other areas of practice (most notably child protection) 'legislation by tabloid' dictated the direction of government policy.

The change process in law and policy

1. Established policy and practice languishes without intervention; 'sleeping dogs are left to lie' with little or no attention.
2. A tragedy occurs or allegations are made about bad practice. The media, seeing itself as the nation's moral guardian, brings it to the public's attention.
3. A 'moral panic' is created, followed by public outrage.
4. Anxiety is raised by interested parties who perceive a 'crisis' and call for investigation and change.
5. Formal inquiries are set up which investigate and make recommendations for change.
6. Practice changes of a major or minor nature, or both, are implemented.
7. The process returns to number 1.

The knee-jerk responses that followed were to have a profound impact on the lives of those in mental distress. These included the introduction of supervision registers to identify and provide information on service users 'who are, or are liable to be, at risk of committing serious violence or suicide, or of serious self neglect' (NHS Management Executive, 1994: 1) and the introduction of the Mental Health (Patients in the Community) Act 1995 which made provision for the supervised discharge of the mentally distressed into the community. Clearly these highly coercive measures were at odds with the philosophies of empowerment and integration and demonstrate starkly the ambiguities inherent in a system that strives to reconcile 'care' and 'control'. As Muijen states, 'the crisis in mental health care has much in common with other value-led issues society has to resolve' (1995: 44). In this sense it is naïve to suggest that the blame for the 'crisis' in community care policy and practice during the 1990s should be laid exclusively at either the door of government of the day or the media. As Barham suggests:

> It needs to be recognised also that some such instabilities and ambiguities are an inevitable, and wholly necessary, consequence of the attempt to overturn traditional ways of disposing of the mentally ill. Deinstitutionalisation implies rather more than the administrative substitution of one locus of care for another, and invites also a drastic reshaping of the ways in which we think about, describe and, in particular, relate to people with a history of mental illness. (1992: 151)

Barham's statement clearly relates to our starting point in Chapter 1 concerning the longstanding persistence of contradictory, alienating and exclusionary attitudes to the mentally distressed in society. The rhetorical acceptance of the mentally distressed into the community has simply not been matched by the conferment of the status of 'citizen' within it – their 'otherness' persists (Sayce, 2000; TNS, 2007). This begs the wider question of whether the community does actually 'care' about, let alone for, the mentally distressed.

On 29 July 1998 the then Health Secretary, Frank Dobson, announced to the House of Commons that 'care in the community has failed'. Rogers and Pilgrim consider this 'an unwise statement', concluding that 'community care had definitely not failed as a policy' (2001: 173). Rather they emphasize how it opened up:

> a new set of debates about the amelioration of distress and dysfunction, the control or tolerance of madness, and the promotion of well being. It also raises a set of questions about citizenship for those who are disabled on a temporary or enduring basis by their mental health problems and the degree to which state-funded services can intervene positively in this regard. (2001: 173)

For Judi Clements (1998) from MIND the issue was straightforward – far from having failed, community care had never really been tried.

NEW LABOUR'S MODERNIZATION OF MENTAL HEALTH SERVICES

Key policy relating to community care for the mentally distressed 1998–2008

1998 The Human Rights Act (effective October 2000)
1998 Modernising Mental Health Services: Safe, Sound and Supportive
1999 Effective Care Co-ordination: Modernising the Care Programme Approach
1999 The National Service Framework for Mental Health: Modern Standards and Service Models
2000 The NHS Plan: A Plan for Investment, a Plan for Reform
2001 The Mental Health Policy Implementation Guide
2001 Shifting the Balance of Power
2002 Shifting the Balance of Power: The next steps
2005 Independence, Well-being and Choice: Our Vision for the Future of Adult Social Care for Adults in England
2005 Your Care, Your Say. Public consultation
2006 Our Health, Our Care, Our Say: A New Direction for Community Services
2007 Putting People First: A Shared Vision and Commitment to the Transformation of Adult Social Care
2007 No Voice, No Choice. Joint Review of Adult Community Mental Health Services

Under the banner of 'safe, sound and supportive' the New Labour government announced its intention to 'modernise' the mental health system (DH, 1998a). In addition to proposals for the reform of mental health legislation (discussed in Chapter 4) a raft of initiatives was set out in the *National Service Framework for Mental Health* published in 1999 and the *NHS Plan* published in 2000. The government also appointed the first ever 'mental health tzar', Louis Appleby. The NSFMH (DH, 1999a) outlined a 10-year programme focused on adults with mental health problems of 'working age' (those between the ages of 18 and 65). It contains seven standards that address different aspects of care:

The National Service Framework for Mental Health

Standard one

Health and social services should:

- promote mental health for all, working with individuals and communities
- combat discrimination against individuals and groups with mental health problems, and promote their social inclusion.

(Continued)

Standard two

Any service user who contacts their primary health care team with a mental health problem should:

- have their mental health needs identified and assessed
- be offered effective treatments, including referral to specialist services for further assessment, treatment and care if they require it.

Standard three

Any individual with a common mental health problem should:

- be able to make contact round the clock with local services necessary to meet their needs and receive adequate care
- be able to use NHS Direct, as it develops, for first-level advice and referral on to specialist helplines or to local services.

Standard four

All mental health service users on CPA should:

- receive care which optimises engagement, anticipates or prevents a crisis, and reduces risk
- have a copy of a written care plan which:
  - includes the action to be taken in a crisis by the service user, their carer, and their care co-ordinator
  - advises their GP how they should respond if the service user needs additional help
  - is regularly reviewed by their care co-ordinator
  - be able to access services 24 hours a day, 365 days a year.

Standard five

Each service user who is assessed as requiring a period of care away from their home should have:

- timely access to an appropriate hospital bed or alternative bed or place, which is:
  - in the least restrictive environment consistent with the need to protect them and the public
  - as close to home as possible
- a copy of a written after care plan agreed on discharge which sets out the care and rehabilitation to be provided, identifies the care co-ordinator, and specifies the action to be taken in a crisis.

Standard six

All individuals who provide regular and substantial care for a person on CPA should:

- have an assessment of their caring, physical and mental health needs, repeated on at least an annual basis
- have their own written care plan which is given to them and implemented in discussion with them.

Standard seven

Local health and social care communities should prevent suicides by:

- support local prison staff in preventing suicides amongst prisoners
- ensure that staff are competent to assess the risk of suicide among individuals at greatest risk
- develop local systems for suicide audit to learn lessons and take any necessary action.

(DH, 1999a)

While the wide-ranging agenda of the NSFMH was generally welcomed, along with its positive sentiments around 'partnership' with and 'choice' for service users, there were nevertheless some reservations – for example: the document was not fully resourced (SCMH, 1999); there was no standard specifically dedicated to service users; and the rhetoric around social inclusion for the mentally distressed was simultaneously being undermined in the proposals for strengthening coercive powers in mental health legislation.

Alongside the NSFMH, *The NHS Plan* (DH, 2000) mapped out an ambitious programme of changes in service delivery and workforce development for the following 10 years including:

- 1,000 new graduate mental health workers in primary care
- an extra 500 staff for community mental health teams
- 50 early intervention teams to provide treatment and support to young people (under 35) with psychosis
- 335 crisis resolution teams
- an increase to 220 assertive outreach teams
- women-only day services
- 700 extra staff to work with carers
- 'more suitable' accommodation for up to 400 people in high security hospitals
- better services for prisoners with mental health problems
- a care plan and key worker for every prisoner leaving prison with serious mental illness.

A *Mental Health Policy Implementation Guide* (DH, 2001a) was also published to support the implementation of the *NHS Plan* and the NSFMH, with detailed descriptions of service models (including crisis resolution; assertive outreach; early intervention; primary care and mental health promotion) and an emphasis on a 'whole systems' approach.

In its first year in office New Labour had published *The New NHS: Modern, Dependable* (DH, 1997) in which, although a commitment was given to abolish the internal market created by the Conservatives, the 'purchaser/provider split' would be retained. The increasing role of primary care in delivering mental health services was reflected in *The New NHS, The NHS Plan* and two subsequent documents, *Shifting the Balance of Power* (DH, 2001b) and *Shifting the Balance of Power: the Next Steps* (DH, 2002a). Primary Care Trusts (PCTs) were acknowledged as the leading NHS organization for partnership with local authorities and other stakeholders, and were eventually given specific responsibility for commissioning all mental health services. The emphasis was now on 'collaboration' and 'partnership' between commissioners and providers rather than competition. Subsequently, there has been a highly complex transition towards integrated Mental Health Care Trusts and Partnership Trusts (with some significant variations in arrangements locally). However, the NHS has more often taken the role of lead agency in the provision of mental health services with the most common model of delivery being the co-location of health and social care staff within community teams. The challenges this poses for effective interprofessional working in mental health are discussed in Chapter 7.

COMMUNITY MENTAL HEALTH TEAMS AND THE MODERN CARE PROGAMME APPROACH

The majority of people in mental distress are now 'cared for' in the community by Community Mental Health Teams (CMHTs). Typically, CMHTs include psychiatrists, mental health nurses, social workers, clinical psychologists and occupational therapists, although, as we discuss in Chapter 7, a variety of new roles have been created in recent years. Psychiatrists, nurses, psychologists and occupational therapists are generally employed by the NHS while social workers are often either seconded from their employing local authority to the 'host' NHS trust (that is they are still employed by the local authority but for operational purposes are responsible to the NHS), or they are employed directly by the trust. These arrangements are not without their problems, particularly for social workers who may face significant changes to their terms and conditions of employment and/or may feel isolated from social work colleagues (NIMHE, 2006). Again this is an issue to which we will return in Chapter 7.

The original confusion created by the overlap in local authority 'care management' and the NHS CPA was technically resolved with the introduction of the NSFMH (DH, 1999a) when both systems were integrated and updated, and revised guidance issued (DH, 1999b). A single care coordination approach was created with health and social services having joint responsibility for appointing a 'lead officer'. The CPA applied to 'all adults of working age in contact with the secondary mental health system (health and social care)' (DH, 1999b: 4) *regardless* of setting (including the community, hospitals, residential care and prisons in the statutory, voluntary and private sectors).

> **The four essential elements of the CPA**
>
> 1. a systematic assessment of health and social care needs
> 2. an agreed care plan
> 3. a named care coordinator
> 4. ongoing review of needs and evaluation of care plan (six monthly).

The revised CPA (DH, 1999b) was in operation from 1999 until October 2008 and service provision operated at two levels – *standard* CPA and *enhanced* CPA – determined through assessment. The distinction between the two levels was made according to the complexity of individual need, the assumption being that the level may change as the needs (and risks) of the individual were subsequently reviewed. The assessment at standard level was essentially the same as that for enhanced CPA, but the main difference was that standard support was for those who only received secondary mental health services from one agency, could manage their mental health problems and maintain contact with services. Enhanced CPA was reserved for those with multiple and complex care needs that necessitated a multi-agency and multidisciplinary approach. Those on enhanced CPA were considered to be at 'higher risk' and 'difficult to engage' with services.

However, resource limitations have dictated that, in practice, only those eligible for enhanced CPA have tended to receive a service. While the Department of Health issues guidance on the CPA, implementation is locally determined through Local Implementation Teams (LITs). In the context of budget constraints and tight expenditure controls this inevitably means that the level and quality of mental health services available can vary considerably – often referred to as the 'postcode' lottery. Mandelstam critically observes that 'notwithstanding the importance of such services, community care is rife with legal and practical uncertainties. Indeed, these uncertainties are so prevalent as to be an integral and essential part of the system' (2005: 36). Furthermore, frustrated practitioners can frequently be heard describing how these 'uncertainties' are routinely exploited by local authorities and NHS trusts to limit their obligations, for example through:

- 'screening people out' in the assessment process
- waiting times for assessment
- setting and varying thresholds of eligibility
- not carrying out full assessments
- placing cost ceilings on care packages
- not providing services that have been assessed as needed
- waiting times for service provision
- cost-shunting between different statutory bodies
- not monitoring and reviewing care packages adequately
- re-assessing needs in order to reduce provision.

These devices are often obscured by the rather cynical use of crude quantitative measures of 'quality' that bear little or no relationship to either service users', carers', or practitioners' real experiences. New Labour's modernization programme has intensified the use of targets and performance monitoring with many practitioners bemoaning the fact that their jobs are dominated by form filling and the amount of time spent on computers, which inevitably drastically reduces the face-to-face relationship work done with service users and carers (Sharkey, 2007). Those practitioners brave enough to speak out about these issues run the risk of disciplinary action or even losing their jobs, as in the case of Karen Reissman, a senior community mental health nurse who was sacked by Manchester Mental Health and Social Care Trust in November 2007 for 'damaging the reputation of the Trust' by publicly criticizing her employer over cuts in mental health care provision.

> I would like to have the time to get to know patients better and build up a relationship with them, but sometimes it's just a cup of tea and a 15-minute chat. It gets frustrating because there's not enough of me or my colleagues to go around. In the past I could take someone shopping for the day but that's gone now. I don't feel that the service properly measures the quality of the care that we give. (cited in the *Observer*, 17 September 2006)

However, it is not just individual mental health practitioners who have expressed ongoing concerns about the gap between the rhetoric and the reality of community care for the mentally distressed. In 2006 two separate investigations by Rethink and the Sainsbury Centre for Mental Health found evidence to suggest that, despite significant extra investment in mental health services between 2001 and 2006, the NHS was 'disinvesting' in, and even diverting money from, mental health services to shore up the balance sheets of over-spending acute hospitals and primary care trusts (Revill, 2006). In the same year the Healthcare Commission reviewed 174 community mental health teams in England and found gaps in out-of-hours care, talking therapies and access to information (Revill, 2006). Only one in 10 CMHTs was rated 'excellent', while almost half only received a 'fair' rating. Chief Executive Anna Walker commented:

> The majority of people who suffer from mental illness receive their treatment in their own community, not in hospital. They want to remain in the community and this helps them get better. But for care in the community to work for the mentally ill, more access is needed to talking therapies and out-of-hours crisis care. Mental health crises don't keep office hours and the service must be flexible enough to tackle this. (*BBC News*, 28 September 2006)

In 2007 the Healthcare Commission identified the need for further improvements to the CPA in relation to meeting the NSFMH standards (CSCI/Healthcare Commission, 2007). It found that:

- many people who used services were not fully involved in decisions about their own care
- too few people were offered or received a written copy of their care plan

- service users were not always aware of who their care coordinator was
- not enough care reviews were taking place
- people needed help with employment.

Subsequently the CPA was subjected to a 'refocusing' exercise in 2008 'to ensure that national policy is more consistently and clearly applied and unnecessary bureaucracy removed' (DH, 2008b: 2). From 1 October 2008 the term 'CPA' is no longer used to describe those receiving standard support. Although no longer eligible for CPA, these service users can nevertheless expect:

- an identified *lead professional*
- that care will be *self-directed*, with support
- a full *assessment of need* including risk
- a care plan in the form of a *statement of care* agreed with them, which will be recorded in notes or a letter
- *on-going review* as required, including the need for inclusion in (new) CPA
- their *carers identified* and informed of their rights to their own assessment
- a short *central record* kept of essential information.

CPA now only applies to 'individuals with a wide range of needs from a number of services, or who are most at risk' (DH, 2008b: 2). These service users can expect:

- the support of a *CPA care coordinator*
- a *comprehensive, multi-disciplinary, multi-agency assessment*
- a comprehensive *formal written care plan* including management of risk and direct payments where appropriate
- formal multidisciplinary, multi-agency *review at least once a year*
- their *carers* identified and informed of their right to their *own assessment*
- increased *advocacy support*.

CPA is now also underpinned by a statement of values and principles.

Statement of values and principles

The approach to individuals' care and support puts them at the centre and promotes *social inclusion and recovery*. It is respectful – building confidence in individuals with an understanding of their strengths, goals and aspirations as well as their needs and difficulties. It recognises the individual as a person first and patient/service user second.

Care assessment and planning views a person *'in the round'* seeing and supporting them in their individual diverse roles and the needs they have, including: family; parenting; relationships; housing; employment; leisure; education; creativity; spirituality; self-management and self-nurture; with the aim of optimising mental and physical health and well-being.

(Continued)

> Self-care is promoted and supported wherever possible. Action is taken to encourage *independence* and *self determination* to help people maintain *control over their own support and care*.
>
> *Carers* form a vital part of the support required to aid a person's recovery. Their own needs should also be *recognised* and *supported*.
>
> Services should be organised and delivered in ways that promote and co-ordinate helpful and purposeful mental health practice based on fulfilling *therapeutic relationships* and *partnerships* between the people involved. These relationships involve shared listening, communicating, understanding, clarification, and organisation of diverse opinion to deliver valued, appropriate, equitable and co-ordinated care. The quality of the relationship between service user and the care co-ordinator is one of the most important determinants of success.
>
> Care planning is underpinned by *long-term engagement*, requiring *trust, team work* and *commitment*. It is the daily work of mental health services and supporting partner agencies, not just the planned occasions where people meet for reviews.
>
> (DH, 2008b: 7, emphasis added)

THE FUTURE FOR COMMUNITY CARE? THE 'PERSONALIZATION AGENDA' AND MENTAL HEALTH

In 2005, the New Labour government embarked upon another radical transformation of public services which began with the public consultation, *Your Care, Your Say* (DH, 2005a), followed by the White Paper, *Our Health, Our Care, Our Say* (DH, 2006) and a Comprehensive Spending Review. These culminated in the publication of a joint Ministerial Concordat with the Local Government Association, NHS, Association of Directors of Adult Social Services and others entitled *Putting People First* (DH, 2007a) and the Local Authority Circular *Transforming Social Care* (DH, 2008c). The proposals aim to meet 'the rising expectations of those who depend on social care for their quality of life and capacity to have full and purposeful lives' (DH, 2007a: 1). The key elements are:

- prevention
- early intervention and re-enablement
- personalization
- information, advice and advocacy

Local authorities are required to move to a system of individual, personalized budgets for everyone who is eligible for publicly funded adult social care support. Moreover, 'everyone who receives social care support, regardless of their level of need … will have choice and control over how that support is delivered' (DH, 2008c: 4). The Department of Health has stated that '"personalization" will be the cornerstone of public services [and] is not a fleeting experiment' (DH, 2008d). Although the reforms are being introduced incrementally the government target is for the process to be completed by March 2011. In addition to the social care reforms, Lord Darzi has been commissioned by the UK government to explore the feasibility of 'personal health budgets' (the NHS equivalent of individual budgets) in relation to a variety of long-term health conditions – including mental health problems.

In the mental health context, statutory services (NHS Trusts and local authority social services departments) have traditionally been in the driving seat of mental health service delivery. However, *Transforming Social Care* (DH, 2008c) envisages the development of a much wider choice of mental health service providers (including service-user-led and voluntary sector organizations) in order that 'choice' and 'control' can become a reality. This implies a profound cultural shift, far beyond that which followed the community care reforms of the 1990s. With its emphasis on user-led outcomes and self-directed care, personalization has the potential to pose a significant challenge to the traditional power relationships between mental health professionals and users of services:

> Professionals will no longer be the holders of all knowledge. Instead, people will be the experts on their own life and condition. We must replace the 'medical model' approach (which defines people wholly by their condition) with person-centred approaches that see the whole person – someone who is an important member of their community. Expert mental health advice and treatment will still be important, but that expertise alone is insufficient. (Brewis, 2008: 1–2)

According to the National Director for Mental Health, Louis Appleby, the refocused CPA 'is at the centre of this personalization focus, supporting individuals with severe mental illness to ensure that their needs and choices remain central in what are often complex systems of care' (DH, 2008b: 1).

Reflection exercise

How do you think the vision of 'personalization' fits with an individual who has a limited, or no grasp of reality? How can such individuals achieve 'choice' and 'control'?

The document *Three Keys to a Shared Approach in Mental Health Assessment* emphasizes the government's goal of 'adapting services to people not people to services' and highlights the challenge 'of achieving personalisation, not only in how services respond to people's problems but also in how their problems are assessed in the first place' (CSIP/NIMHE, 2008: 2). It recognizes that person-centred services depend on person-centred assessments 'that are carried out in ways that make sense to the person concerned and that build strongly on their strengths and aspirations as well as aiming to understand their needs and difficulties' (2008: 3). Moreover, it acknowledges that such assessments are underpinned by *genuinely shared approaches* between practitioners, people who use services, and their carers.

> ### The three keys to the shared approach
>
> 1. *active participation* of the service user concerned in a shared understanding with service providers and where appropriate with their carers
> 2. input from *different provider perspectives* within a multidisciplinary approach, and
> 3. a person-centred focus that builds on the *strengths, resiliencies and aspirations* of the individual service user as well as identifying his or her needs and challenges.
>
> (CSIP/NIMHE, 2008: 4, original emphases)

The powerful positive rhetoric of personalization or person-centred support is that it will offer service users greater choice and control, but it must be recognized that these concepts are particularly problematic in relation to users of mental health services. They imply a level of personal autonomy and self-determination that is fundamentally at odds with the philosophy of the current mental health system – a system that is essentially characterized by both authoritarian risk-aversion and disabling paternalism. There can be no underestimation of the scale of cultural shift in the mental health field that will be required in order to bring about genuine choice and control for users of mental health services. It will need to involve 'a new approach based on enabling people to take positive risks rather than always stopping them doing things because the authorities could see risks involved for them. And it would require real ongoing user involvement at every level, from top to bottom, for each individual service user and to make possible a properly resourced network of user controlled organizations' (Beresford, 2008: 7).

It is early days for the personalization agenda and it remains to be seen whether the rhetoric will be matched in reality. By the end of 2008 there were already some worrying signs that the original political enthusiasm for personalization may be waning. The economic climate has changed significantly since the reforms were first announced and subsequent events may jeopardize the progress towards achieving the original aims. As Beresford argues:

> This wouldn't be the first time that a pioneering development in social care got lost through failures in top-down implementation. We saw it with patch social work and indeed care management. Some key steps are now needed if person-centred support and individual budgets are to succeed at ground level. Policymakers must engage with, help and support the face-to-face practitioners who have the key role to play in taking personalisation forward. They must connect better with the wide range of service users who could truly benefit from individual budgets. IBs have got to be put into place

with a proper infrastructure of support for service users, including information, advice, advocacy and administrative back-up, plus proper resourcing and capacity-building for staff. Then we may see those real moves to independent living we were promised – for *all* service users and particularly from our point of view for mental health service users. (2008: 8–9)

CHAPTER SUMMARY

In 1999 Bartlett and Wright argued that 'in the closing years of the twentieth century "care in the community" holds the dubious distinction of being universally supported in principle, and universally condemned in practice'. They reflected that there was much to condemn: 'Chronic underfunding from governments, poor co-ordination of service providers at the local level, rivalry among professional bodies, lack of continuity of care and a general misunderstanding and resistance by the public ... inherent in this contested programme of social engineering' (1999: 16).

It would be unfair to suggest that nothing has improved for people in mental distress in the community since that time. Many people have been and are supported at home by committed, hard-working mental health professionals in community teams. Indeed a recent World Health Organization Report (WHO, 2008) showed England's mental health services to be among the best in Europe, with higher levels of investment than in any other country. With its 700 community mental health teams, it is one of only three states to offer home treatment to most service users. Social workers specializing in mental health receive up to 400 undergraduate training hours in mental health, the second highest in Europe. However, the report also showed that there was still room for improvement.

Clearly, the objectives of community care are still to be fully realized and whether the ongoing reorganizations in health and social care policy and practice will create seamless and effective care remains to be seen. Despite the many policy initiatives outlined in this chapter, as Boardman argues, 'areas such as mental health promotion, primary care services and rehabilitation remain poorly developed (possibly as a consequence of the focus on acute care associated with the emphasis on control)' (2005: 34). In a number of ways the original aims of community care remain obscured, with Mandelstam arguing that instead of being straightforward 'a system has developed that is generally characterized by extraordinary contortion and complexity' (2005: 39). At the same time neo-liberal ideology and politics has corrupted much of the original person-centred philosophies of community care. For example, notions of 'care' which include 'standing on your own two feet' and not involving the 'nanny state' are limiting when offering social work assistance to those in mental distress in the community. Similarly, the ambiguities and conflicts surrounding the 'rights' of the mentally distressed to 'care' and 'support' in the community versus the 'rights' of the public for protection from 'such people' are far from reconciled. These enduring tensions and contradictions lie at the heart of policy and practice in mental health.

Further reading/resources

Carr, S. (2008) *SCIE Report 20: Personalisation: a Rough Guide*. London: SCIE.
Salter, M. and Turner, T. (2007) *Community Mental Health Care: a Practical Guide to Outdoor Psychiatry*. Oxford: Churchill Livingstone.
Sharkey, P. (2007) *The Essentials of Community Care*, 2nd edn. Basingstoke: Palgrave Macmillan.
www.carersuk.org – Carers UK.
www.mind.org.uk – the National Association for Mental Health.
www.spn.org.uk – the Social Perspectives Network for Modern Mental Health.

4

RISK VERSUS RIGHTS

The tensions in implementing mental health law

This chapter can be used to support the development of knowledge and skills in professional social work as follows:

National Occupational Standards for Social Work

Key Role 1: Prepare for, and work with individuals, families, carers, groups and communities to assess their needs and circumstances

- Prepare for social work contact and involvement.

Key Role 2: Plan, carry out, review and evaluate social work practice, with individuals, families, carers, groups and communities and other professionals

- Respond to crisis situations
- Address behaviour which presents a risk to individuals, families, carers, groups, communities.

Key Role 3: Support individuals to represent their needs, views and circumstances

- Prepare for, and participate in decision making forums.

Key Role 4: Manage risk to individuals, families, carers, groups, communities, self and colleagues

- Assess and manage risks to individuals, families, carers, groups and communities
- Assess, minimise and manage risk to self and colleagues.

Key Role 5: Manage and be accountable, with supervision and support, for your own social work practice within your organisation

- Work within multi-disciplinary and multi-organisational teams, networks and systems.

Key Role 6: Demonstrate professional competence in social work practice

- Managing complex ethical issues, dilemmas and conflicts.

(TOPPS England, 2002)

Academic Standards for Social Work

Honours graduates in social work:

4.4 should be equipped to understand, and to work within, the context of contested debate about the nature, scope and purpose of social work.

5.1 should acquire, critically evaluate, apply and integrate knowledge and understanding in relation to:

5.1.1 Social work services, service users and carers

- the relationship between agency policies, legal requirements and professional boundaries in shaping the nature of services provided in interdisciplinary contexts and the issues associated with working across professional boundaries and within different disciplinary groups.

5.1.2 The service delivery context

- the significance of legislative and legal frameworks and service delivery standards (including the nature of legal authority, the application of legislation in practice, statutory accountability and tensions between statute, policy and practice).

5.1.3 Values and ethics

- the moral concepts of rights, responsibility, freedom, authority and power inherent in the practice of social workers as moral and statutory agents
- the complex relationships between justice, care and control in social welfare and the practical and ethical implications of these, including roles as statutory agents and in upholding the law in respect of discrimination.

5.1.4 Social work theory

- models and methods of assessment, including factors underpinning the selection and testing of relevant information, the nature of professional judgement and the process of risk assessment and decision-making.

(QAA, 2008)

Key themes in this chapter

- The statutory context for modern mental health practice
- The 'sectioning' process and arrangements governing the use of compulsory powers in mental health practice
- The role of the AMHP
- Theorizing risk in mental health practice
- The politics of compulsory detention and treatment
- The Human Rights Act 1998
- The centrality of values and ethics in implementing mental health law.

INTRODUCTION

History has demonstrated that the legal aspects surrounding mental distress are not straightforward. Each piece of legislation arises from the policy agendas and government priorities of its day and so is liable to the perpetual round of revision and change. As Rogers and Pilgrim note:

> Mental health policy refers to legal arrangements, policy directives and service investments. It is partly about the control of mad behaviour, partly about promoting well-being, partly about ameliorating distress and partly about responding to dysfunction. Given such a wide remit it is hardly surprising that the notion of mental health policy is now highly ambiguous. A century ago such an ambiguity did not exist: there was basically *a lunacy policy,* with segregation (the asylum system) being the single total organisational solution. (2001: 226)

Moreover, there is not only mental health law itself, but also guidance frameworks and codes of practice for the *implementation* of such law. The law attempts to strike a difficult balance between the rights of an individual, the rights of that individual's family/carers and the overall protection of society. For practitioners, the implementation of the law can be fraught with tension, arising from the inherent ambiguities and contradictions that inevitably follow when attempting to balance such conflicting interests. In the modern mental health system it is a balancing act that involves both the assessment and management of 'risk'. For social workers to practise effectively and legally in the modern mental health system they need to be fully informed; which includes an awareness of the relationship between human rights and mental health law. It is not the intention of this chapter to cover every aspect of this complex area of practice, but to address some of the key issues relating to risks, rights, responsibilities and the centrality of values and ethics in implementing mental health law.

THE STATUTORY CONTEXT FOR MODERN MENTAL HEALTH PRACTICE

The majority of people receiving in-patient psychiatric care and treatment are *informal patients*. This means they are in hospital on a *voluntary* basis and they have exactly the same rights as a person being treated for a physical illness. About one-fifth of psychiatric in patients are *formal patients*. These are persons who are *compulsorily* detained under a section of the Mental Health Act 1983. As a consequence of being 'sectioned' these people lose some of the rights available to informal patients. This chapter outlines some of the main provisions of the Mental Health Act 1983 as they affect formal patients and their relatives.

The Mental Health Act 1983 (MHA 1983) has undergone several amendments since its first implementation, and the discussion here incorporates those amendments. At the time of writing the latest amendments are those introduced with the passing of the Mental Health Act 2007 (MHA 2007), the main provisions of which came into effect from 3 November 2008. The MHA 2007 was also used to introduce 'deprivation of liberty safeguards' (DoLS) through amending the Mental Capacity Act 2005 (MCA 2005), and to extend the rights of victims by amending the Domestic Violence, Crime and Victims Act 2004. It should also be remembered that, in practice, the MHA 1983 operates in conjunction with other relevant legislation such as the Human Rights Act 1998 (HRA 1998) and the NHS and Community Care Act 1990 (NHSCCA 1990).

MENTAL HEALTH ACT 1983

In 1998 the New Labour government announced a major review of the MHA 1983 and brought forward proposals for a new Mental Health Act. These proposals proved highly controversial, attracting widespread opposition from the Mental Health Alliance – an alliance of mental health organizations, practitioners, service users and carers. After almost 10 years of heated debate and political wrangling the government was forced to abandon plans for a new Act and instead opted to amend the MHA 1983. The MHA 2007 received Royal Assent on 19 July 2007 and became law on 3 November 2008. The bulk of the MHA 1983 remained intact but with some significant amendments. According to the government:

> The main purpose of the legislation is to ensure that people with serious mental disorders which threaten their health or safety or the safety of the public can be treated irrespective of their consent where it is necessary to prevent them from harming themselves or others. (DH, 2007b)

The *Reference Guide to the Mental Health Act 1983* (DH, 2008e) explains the provisions of the MHA 1983 as amended by the MHA 2007. However, it should be noted that:

> it is not intended as a complete description of every aspect of the Act and must not be relied on as a definitive statement of the law. It is not a substitute for consulting the Act itself or for taking legal advice. Guidance on the way the Act should be applied to practice is given in the Code of Practice. (DH, 2008e: 15)

The MHA 1983 is accompanied by a revised *Code of Practice* (DH, 2008f) which gives detailed guidance on implementation of the law in practice. Though it is deemed good practice to follow the Code it is not binding in law as it is for *guidance* rather than instruction. Despite strong campaigning by the Mental Health Alliance, the Government refused to use the MHA 2007 to introduce fundamental principles to the MHA 1983 itself. Instead, the revised *Code of Practice* sets out five guiding principles that should be considered when making decisions about a course of action under the Act.

> **The five guiding principles**
>
> Purpose principle
>
> Decisions under the Act must be taken with a view to minimising the undesirable effects of mental disorder, by maximising the safety and wellbeing (mental and physical) of patients, promoting their recovery and protecting other people from harm.
>
> Least restriction principle
>
> People taking action without a patient's consent must attempt to keep to a minimum the restrictions they impose on the patient's liberty, having regard to the purpose for which the restrictions are imposed.
>
> Respect principle
>
> People taking decisions under the Act must recognise and respect the diverse needs, values and circumstances of each patient, including their race, religion, culture, gender, age, sexual orientation and any disability. They must consider the patient's views, wishes and feelings (whether expressed at the time or in advance), so far as they are reasonably ascertainable, and follow those wishes wherever practicable and consistent with the purpose of the decision. There must be no unlawful discrimination.
>
> Participation principle
>
> Patients must be given the opportunity to be involved, as far as is practicable in the circumstances, in planning, developing and reviewing their own treatment and care to help ensure that it is delivered in a way that is as appropriate and effective for them as possible. The involvement of carers, family members and other people who have an interest in the patient's welfare should be encouraged (unless there are particular reasons to the contrary) and their views taken seriously.
>
> Effectiveness, efficiency and equity principle
>
> People taking decisions under the Act must seek to use the resources available to them and to patients in the most effective and equitable way, to meet the needs of patients and achieve the purpose for which the decision was taken.
>
> (DH, 2008f: 5–6)

DEFINITION OF MENTAL DISORDER

As initially discussed in Chapter 1, the terminology surrounding mental 'health' and mental 'illness' can be problematic. This is particularly significant in relation to mental health law where there has never been a unified definition of the term 'mental illness'. However, the MHA 2007 changed the way the MHA 1983 defines 'mental disorder' so that a single definition applies throughout the Act – 'any disorder or disability of the mind' – and abolished references to categories of disorder. It should be noted that a person with a learning disability is not considered to be suffering from mental disorder for most purposes under the Act, or to require treatment in hospital, unless that disability is associated with abnormally aggressive or seriously irresponsible conduct.

KEY ROLES

Approved Mental Health Practitioner (AMHP)

The AMHP role is newly created in the MHA 2007 and replaces that of the Approved Social Worker. Whereas previously only social workers could be Approved Social Workers, an AMHP may be a social worker, nurse, occupational therapist or psychologist. Approved Mental Health Practitioners are approved by a local social services authority (LSSA) to carry out certain functions under the MHA 1983. The MHA 1983 gives the AMHP the power to make an application for admission to hospital under a section of the Act. However, before any application is made, the AMHP must interview the patient and satisfy him or herself that detention in hospital is, in all the circumstances, the most appropriate way of providing the care and medical treatment the patient needs. The role of the AMHP is discussed more fully later in the chapter.

Approved Clinician (AC)

This is a new role introduced in the MHA 2007. Some functions under the MHA 1983 that were formerly only assigned to a registered medical practitioner can now be undertaken by an approved clinician, for example the 'holding power' to detain a patient already in hospital for up to 72 hours. The approved clinician is a mental health professional who has been approved, for the purposes of the Act, by the Secretary of State (England) or by Welsh ministers (Wales). The approved clinician is expected to be competent to undertake mental health assessments, understand the range of treatment options available and their applicability to patients, and to lead a multi-disciplinary team. Approved clinicians may be doctors or non-medically qualified mental health professionals such as psychologists, nurses, occupational therapists and social workers. However, certain functions under the MHA 1983 will still require the input of a medical doctor. The wording of sections 2 and 3, for instance, still require medical recommendations for detention under these sections to be made by two registered medical practitioners.

Responsible Clinician (RC)

This is another new role introduced in the MHA 2007 and replaces that of the Responsible Medical Officer who previously held full legal and clinical responsibility for detained patients. A responsible clinician is the approved clinician with overall responsibility for a patient's care and treatment. Certain decisions, such as placing a detained patient on supervised community treatment, can only be taken by the RC. The responsible clinician does not need to be a medical doctor but all responsible clinicians must be Approved Clinicians (as outlined above).

Nearest Relative (NR)

The nearest relative holds an important role in terms of admission, care and discharge of a patient. The nearest relative can apply for their relative to be formally detained under a section of the Act, but in the vast majority of cases it is an AMHP who makes an application. The NR role is determined on the basis of priority on the list of relatives listed in section 26 of the Act as follows:

- spouse (disregarded if separated, and a cohabite of 6 months or more is treated as a spouse)
- son/daughter
- parent
- sibling
- grandparent
- grandchild
- uncle/aunt
- nephew/niece.

Priority is given to a person on the list who cares for the patient. In addition any other person with whom the patient resides and has done for five years can also be treated as a relative. This is not the same as next of kin. The NR must be consulted before an application for treatment or guardianship is made and if the NR objects the application will not proceed. The MHA 2007 gives patients the right to make an application to displace their nearest relative and enables County Courts to displace a NR where there are reasonable grounds for doing so (section 29). The provisions for determining the NR were amended to include civil partners amongst the list of relatives.

Hospital Managers

The hospital managers are legally responsible for patients detained under the MHA 1983. They are required to ensure that the patient's treatment and care and all documentation relating to the patient's detention is consistent with the specific section under which they have been detained. They must ensure that the patient is not only informed of their rights, but also (as far as possible) *understands* their rights.

Independent Mental Health Advocates (IMHA)

The role of Independent Mental Health Advocate was introduced in the MHA 2007, and they are specially trained advocates. 'Qualifying' patients (defined under section 130C of the Act) are entitled to help from IMHAs which may include help in obtaining information relating to their detention, treatment and rights under the MHA 1983.

Best Interests Assessor (BIA)

In response to the 2004 European Court of Human Rights judgement (HL v UK (Application No.45508/99)) (the 'Bournewood judgement'), involving an autistic man who was kept at Bournewood Hospital by doctors against the wishes of his carers, the MHA 2007 amended the MCA 2005 and made provision for procedures authorizing the deprivation of the liberty of a person resident in a hospital or care home who lacks capacity to consent. The new role of Best Interests Assessor was created to ensure that any act or decision made for or on behalf of a person who lacks capacity is made in their best interests. Additionally, Deprivation of Liberty Safeguards (DoLS) were introduced. The principle of supporting a person to make a decision when possible, and acting at all times in the least restrictive manner, applies to all decision-making.

The Mental Health Review Tribunal (MHRT)

The MHRT is an independent body that operates under the provisions of the MHA 1983. Its main purpose is to review the cases of patients detained under the MHA 1983 and to direct the discharge of any patients where the statutory criteria for discharge have been satisfied. In some cases the MHRT has the discretion to discharge patients who do not meet the requirements. Such cases usually involve a balanced judgement on a number of serious issues such as the freedom of the individual, the protection of the public and the best interests of the patient. The Council on Tribunals governs MHRTs and the Department of Health administers them regionally. Tribunal hearings are normally held in private. Each MHRT sits with three members – a lawyer, a psychiatrist and a lay person. The principal powers of a MHRT are:

- to discharge a detained patient from hospital immediately or after a further short period of detention
- to recommend leave of absence
- to recommend Supervised Community Treatment
- to recommend transfer to another hospital.

Patients are entitled to be represented at the Tribunal by a solicitor with specialist mental health experience whose services are free under the legal aid scheme. A social circumstances report may be required from a social worker who does not have to be an AMHP.

Mental Health Act Commission (MHAC)

The Mental Health Act Commission provides a safeguard for people who are detained in hospital under the powers of the MHA 1983. The Commission is a monitoring body rather than an inspectorate or regulator. Its concern is primarily the legality of detention and the protection of individuals' human rights. Its functions are:

- to keep under review the operation of the Mental Health Act 1983 in respect of patients detained or liable to be detained under that Act.
- to visit and interview, in private, patients detained under the Mental Health Act in hospitals and mental nursing homes.
- to consider the investigation of complaints where these fall within the Commission's remit.
- to review decisions to withhold the mail of patients detained in the high security hospitals.
- to appoint registered medical practitioners and others to give second opinions in cases where this is required by the Mental Health Act.
- to publish and lay before Parliament a report every two years
- to monitor the implementation of the Code of Practice and propose amendments to Ministers.

The MHAC comprises approximately 100 part-time commissioners: mainly lawyers and mental health professionals, but also some service users. Their functions are expected to be transferred to the Care Quality Commission in 2009.

THE SECTIONING PROCESS

The term being 'sectioned' refers to the use of a section of the MHA 1983 to compulsorily detain a person against their will. The revised *Code of Practice* (DH, 2008f) sets out the grounds for applying for detention. It states:

> Before it is decided that admission to hospital is necessary; consideration must be given to whether there are alternative means of providing the care and treatment which the patient requires. This includes consideration of whether there might be other effective forms of care or treatment which the patient would be willing to accept, and of whether guardianship would be appropriate instead. (DH, 2008f: para 4.4)

and in (para 4.5):

> In all cases, consideration must be given to:
> - the patient's wishes and view of their own needs;
> - the patient's age and physical health;
> - any past wishes or feelings expressed by the patient;
> - the patient's cultural background
> - the patient's social and family circumstances;

- the impact that any future deterioration or lack of improvement in the patient's condition would have on their children, other relatives or carers, especially those living with the patient, including an assessment of these people's ability and willingness to cope; and
- the effect on the patient, and those close to the patient, of a decision to admit or not to admit under the Act.

After consideration of all possible alternative means of providing care, it may be necessary for an individual to be detained under a compulsory order in a hospital. Application for compulsory admission is made to the proposed hospital managers and is accompanied by the power to convey the person to hospital.

The main provisions of the MHA 1983 relating to admission to hospital

Section 2. Admission for assessment

Duration of detention: 28 days maximum.
Application for admission: by an AMHP or the patient's nearest relative. The applicant must have seen the patient within the previous 14 days.
Procedure: two doctors must confirm that

(a) the patient is suffering from a mental disorder of a nature or degree that warrants detention in hospital for assessment (or assessment followed by medical treatment) for at least a limited period; *and*
(b) he or she ought to be detained in the interests of his or her own health or safety, or with a view to the protection of others.

Discharge: by any of the following

- responsible clinician
- hospital managers
- the nearest relative, who must give 72 hours' notice. The responsible clinician can prevent him or her discharging a patient by making a report to the hospital managers
- MHRT. The patient can apply to a tribunal within the first 14 days of detention.

Section 3. Admission for treatment

Duration of detention: up to six months, renewable for a further six months, then for one year at a time.
Application for admission: by nearest relative, or AMHP in cases where the nearest relative does not object, or is displaced by County Court, or it is not 'reasonably practicable' to consult him or her.
Procedure: two doctors must confirm that

(a) the patient is suffering from a mental disorder (see above) of a nature or degree that makes it appropriate for him or her to receive medical treatment in hospital; *and*

(b) appropriate medical treatment is available for him or her; *and*
(c) it is necessary for his or her own health or safety, or for the protection of others that he or she receives such treatment and it cannot be provided unless he or she is detained under this section.

Renewal: under section 20, the responsible clinician can renew a section 3 detention if the original criteria still apply and appropriate medical treatment is available for the patient's condition. If the responsible clinician is not a registered medical practitioner, he or she must consult another person who has been professionally concerned with the patient's treatment, who may be, but does not need to be, a qualified medical practitioner.

Discharge: by any of the following

- responsible clinician
- hospital managers
- the nearest relative, who must give 72 hours' notice. If the responsible clinician prevents the nearest relative discharging the patient, by making a report to the hospital managers, the nearest relative can apply to an MHRT within 28 days
- MHRT. A patient can apply to a tribunal once during the first six months of his or her detention, once during the second six months and then once during each period of one year. If the patient does not apply in the first six months of detention, his or her case will be referred, automatically, to the MHRT. After that, the case is automatically referred when a period of three years has passed since a tribunal last considered it (one year, if the patient is under 16).

Section 4. Admission for assessment in cases of emergency

Duration of detention: 72 hours maximum.
Application for admission: by an AMHP or the nearest relative. The applicant must have seen the patient within the previous 24 hours.
Procedure: one doctor must confirm that

(a) it is of 'urgent necessity' for the patient to be admitted and detained under section 2; *and*
(b) waiting for a second doctor to confirm the need for an admission under section 2 would cause 'undesirable delay'.

Note: the patient must be admitted within 24 hours of the medical examination or application, whichever is the earlier, or the application under section 4 is null and void.

Section 5. Compulsory detention of informal patients already in hospital

A doctor or other approved clinician in charge of an informal patient's treatment (including inpatients being treated for a physical problem), can detain a patient for up to 72 hours by reporting to hospital managers that an application for compulsory admission 'ought to be made'.

A nurse of the prescribed class (a nurse trained to work with mental illness or learning disabilities) can detain an informal patient who is receiving treatment for mental disorder

(Continued)

> for up to six hours, or until a doctor or a clinician with authority to detain him or her arrives, whichever is earlier ...
>
> ### Section 135. Warrant to search for and remove patients
>
> **Duration of detention**: 72 hours maximum.
> **Procedure**: if there is reasonable cause to suspect that a person is suffering from mental disorder *and*
>
> (a) is being ill-treated or neglected or not kept under proper control; *or*
> (b) is unable to care for him or herself and lives alone a magistrate can issue a warrant authorising a police officer (with a doctor and AMHP) to enter any premises where the person is believed to be and remove him or her to a place of safety.
>
> ### Section 136. Mentally disordered persons found in public places
>
> **Duration of detention**: 72 hours maximum.
> **Procedure**: if it appears to a police officer that a person in a public place is 'suffering from mental disorder' and is 'in immediate need of care or control', he or she can take that person to a 'place of safety', which is usually a hospital, but can be a police station. Section 136 lasts for a maximum of 72 hours, so that the person can be examined by a doctor and interviewed by an AMHP and 'any necessary arrangements' made for his or her treatment or care.
>
> (MIND, 2008a)

COMPULSORY POWERS IN THE COMMUNITY

Guardianship

Applying only to patients over the age of 16, guardianship provides a limited amount of control and support for patients who remain in the community. Guardianship orders can be either a civil process (applied for by a NR or AMHP) or can be made through the courts. The criteria for the use of guardianship are set out in section 7 of the Act as follows:

> ... the person is suffering from a mental disorder, being mental illness, severe mental impairment, psychopathic disorder or mental impairment and it is of a nature or degree that warrants reception into guardianship, and it is necessary in the interest of the welfare of the patient or for the protection of others that the patient be received.

The powers of the guardian are set out in section 8 as follows:

a) to require the patient to live in a place specified by the guardian
b) to require the patient to attend at specified places for medical treatment, occupation, education or training
c) to require access to the patient to be given at the place where he is living to any registered medical practitioner, AMHP or other specified person.

Guardianship is initially for six months with the possibility for renewals.

Supervised Community Treatment (SCT)

Controversially, the MHA 2007 introduced Supervised Community Treatment (SCT) for the first time – an arrangement where a patient is discharged from detention in hospital under the MHA 1983 but is required to comply with conditions set out in a Community Treatment Order (CTO) as a 'community patient'; otherwise he or she may be recalled to hospital for treatment. The government's stated intention in introducing SCT was to address the situation whereby some patients leave hospital and do not continue with their treatment, their health deteriorates and they require detention again, thus creating the so-called 'revolving door'. It is argued that SCT will enable these patients to live in the community whilst subject to certain conditions under the MHA 1983 to ensure that they continue with the medical treatment they need. However, many mental health practitioners, service users and carers are fundamentally opposed to SCT as will be discussed later in this chapter.

THE ROLE OF THE APPROVED MENTAL HEALTH PRACTITIONER

While the responsibilities and tasks of the AMHP largely stay the same as those of the former ASW, AMHPs, unlike ASWs, do not have to be qualified social workers. This major change has caused great anxiety for many mental health social workers, service users and carers, especially regarding the capacity of other professionals to maintain the necessary objectivity and independence from the medical model that has been the foundation of the ASW role to date. Furthermore, unlike social work practitioners, the training and practice of these other professionals are not necessarily based on social justice principles. We will return to these concerns in Chapter 7.

Reflection exercise

What do you think are the potential advantages and disadvantages of other professionals now taking on the traditional ASW role?

The *Reference Guide to the Mental Health Act 1983* (DH, 2008e) lists the people who can apply to become an AMHP:

- social workers registered with the General Social Care Council (GSCC)
- registered first-level nurses whose field of practice is mental health nursing or learning disabilities nursing
- registered occupational therapists
- chartered psychologists who hold a relevant practising certificate issued by the British Psychological Society.

Section 114(2) specifically prohibits doctors being approved as AMHPs. Existing ASWs are automatically treated as having been approved as an AMHP for the remaining period of their approval.

An AMHP can be employed by a local social services authority (LSSA), an NHS trust or even be self-employed. Approval to practise as an AMHP is given by a LSSA following completion of an approved AMHP training course recognized by the GSCC. In awarding approval the LSSA must be satisfied that the person has appropriate competence in dealing with people who are suffering from mental disorder and take into account five key competencies related to the applicant, which are:

- application of values to the AMHP role
- application of knowledge – the legal and policy framework
- application of knowledge – mental disorder
- application of skills – working in partnership
- application of skills – making and communicating informed decisions.

The LSSA must also ensure that candidates satisfy the 'Key Competencies' for approval (set out in Schedule 2 of the AMHP Regulations). Approval is conditional on an AMHP completing at least 18 hours of training in the year, starting with the day of their approval, and in each subsequent year. The training must be agreed with the approving LSSA.

The main functions of the Approved Mental Health Professional

- Making applications for admission to hospital for assessment or treatment under Part 2 of the *MHA 1983*.
- The power to convey patients to hospital on the basis of applications for admission.
- Making applications for guardianship.
- Providing social circumstances reports on patients detained on the basis of an application for admission made by their nearest relative.
- Applying to the county court for the replacement of an unsatisfactory private guardian.
- Confirming that community treatment orders (CTOs) should be made discharging patients from detention in hospital on to supervised community treatment (SCT) and agreeing the conditions to be included in the CTO.
- Approving the extensions of CTOs.
- Approving the revocation of CTOs.
- Being consulted by responsible clinicians before they make reports confirming the detention or SCT of patients who have been absent without leave for more than 28 days.
- Applying to the county court for the appointment of an acting nearest relative and the displacement of an existing nearest relative.
- Having the right to enter and inspect premises under section 115.
- Applying for warrants to enter premises under section 135.
- The power to take patients into custody and take them to the place they ought to be when they have gone absent without leave (AWOL).
- The power to take and return other patients who have absconded.

(DH, 2008e: 259)

THEORIZING RISK IN MENTAL HEALTH PRACTICE

In considering detention and compulsory treatment, risks need to be balanced between the safety of the patient and the protection of 'others' – in political terms this is usually taken to mean the general public. The Department of Health identifies 'risk management' as 'a core component of mental health care and the Care Programme Approach' (DH, 2007b: 7). Guidance on risk management can be found in two main government sources – the revised *Code of Practice* to the MHA 1983 (DH, 2008f) and *Best Practice in Managing Risk* (DH, 2007b).

> **Factors to consider**
>
> ### The health or safety of the patient
>
> Factors to be considered in deciding whether patients should be detained for their own health or safety include:
>
> - the evidence suggesting that patients are at risk of:
>   - suicide;
>   - self-harm;
>   - self-neglect or being unable to look after their own health or safety; or
>   - jeopardizing their own health or safety accidentally, recklessly or unintentionally; or that their mental disorder is otherwise putting their health or safety at risk;
> - any evidence suggesting that the patient's mental health will deteriorate if they do not receive treatment;
> - the reliability of such evidence, including what is known of the history of the patient's mental disorder;
> - the views of the patient and of any carers, relatives or close friends, especially those living with the patient, about the likely course of the disorder and the possibility of it improving;
> - the patient's own skills and experience in managing their condition
> - the potential benefits of treatment, which should be weighed against any adverse effects that being detained might have on the patient's well being; and
> - whether other methods of managing the risk are available.
>
> ### Protection of others
>
> In considering whether detention is necessary for the protection of other people, the factors to consider are, the nature of the risk to other people arising from the patient's mental disorder, the likelihood that harm will result and the severity of any potential harm, taking into account:
>
> - that it is not always possible to differentiate risk of harm to the patient from the risk of harm to others;
>
> *(Continued)*

- the reliability of the available evidence, including any relevant details of the patient's clinical history and past behaviour, such as contact with other agencies and (where relevant) criminal convictions and cautions;
- the willingness and ability of those who live with the patient and those who provide care and support to the patient to cope with and manage the risk
- whether other methods of managing the risk are available.

Harm to other people includes psychological as well as physical harm.

(DH, 2008f: 26–7)

Case study

The police have been called to Harry who has armed himself with a hammer and a knife. The police see Harry as a risk to others. Harry says they are to defend himself against attack from others. There appears to be no evidence of a possible attack. How should an AMHP proceed when called to assist?

In the foreword to *Best Practice in Managing Risk*, National Director for Mental Health, Louis Appleby comments:

> it is unrealistic to expect services to prevent all deaths, but the clinical management of risk can be strengthened. We know that an unacceptable number of patients who die by suicide or commit homicide have not been subject to enhanced CPA, despite indications of risk. We also know that staff sometimes feel unable to intervene to reduce risk, feeling that tragedies are inevitable. (DH, 2007b: 3)

The document is intended to guide mental health practitioners who work with service users to manage the risk of harm, and states that: 'organizations, care teams and individual practitioners should benchmark their current practice against the principles set out here' (DH, 2007b: 4). Sixteen best practice points for effective risk management are identified which are grouped into:

- fundamentals
- basic ideas in risk management
- working with service users and carers
- individual practice and team working.

Three main areas of risk are dealt with:

- violence (including anti-social and offending behaviour)
- self harm/suicide
- self neglect.

In an effort to address the question of what constitutes best practice for conducting risk management in these areas the Appendix contains 'tools' that can guide risk decision-making. Some of these tools 'are deliberately designed to predict risk – often in specific groups' and while 'positive risk management' is recommended, it is nevertheless acknowledged, 'that risk can never be completely eliminated' (DH, 2007b: 7, 10).

Many professionals, such as those in the emergency services, deal with 'risk' on a daily basis, and a wide literature exists on this. Dealing with/responding to risk situations is also part of the social work task and too often it places workers in the glare of the media, especially when someone is seriously hurt or dies. Assessment of risk frequently takes centre stage in decision-making about mental health issues, essentially because life and death may be involved, which in itself can make it a stressful exercise for professional social workers. Alaszewski et al. comment that 'front line workers often contend that their job is nothing more than the "management of risk", having to "make risk judgements" and "take risky decisions"' (quoted in Webb, 2006: 66). However, unlike others dealing with life emergencies, social workers are not thanked for trying if they fail in their attempts to save life.

Drawing on Ryan, Kemshall argues that risk itself is a 'contested' area, and 'while community care and risk taking have emphasized client needs and rights, in reality mental health risks have been increasingly negatively defined and community care has become focused on how to increase compliance with community treatments and surveillance' (2002: 93). Thus, she argues that 'community care has become preoccupied with risk avoidance and risk management, resulting in a largely negative view of user risks and a deprioritizing of user rights' (2002: 93). Although the notion of 'risk' is overwhelmingly discussed in mental health services in relation to the risk posed by the patient's behaviour, Vassilev and Pilgrim argue that 'it is actually a two way process. Psychiatric patients are often detained without trial so they always risk losing their liberty' (2007: 352).

Moreover, while the risks involved of a man running amok in a city centre wielding a samurai sword are somewhat easier to define and deal with, assessing the risks involved with the danger of 'psychological harm' as well as physical harm is more complicated. Stephen Webb (2006) likens the work of social workers in this area to that of an insurance actuary who calculates the probability of risk for an insurance company, and refers to this as the rise of 'actuarialism' in social work; a social insurance against risk. Within the caring professions actuarialism is dependent upon the new technologies of computer assisted integrated assessment, decision analysis, information management, evidence-based practice and risk evaluation. Inevitably time spent in these areas drastically reduces the face-to-face relationship work done with service users. On returning to practice Sharkey (2007) notes his surprise at the daunting amount of form filling and the amount of time spent on computers, while the dilemmas, problems and crises of service users continue to exist and require an appropriate human response.

Lupton argues that 'the identification of 'risks' takes place in the specific sociocultural and historical contexts in which we are located', and notes the shift from the concept of 'dangerousness' to that of 'risk' (1999: 13). Nineteenth-century governmental discourses on marginalized social groups and individuals identified 'dangerous classes' and 'dangerous individuals' – dangerous to the more socially and economically privileged, who were seen to be 'at risk' from their depravations or from contamination. Castel comments that:

> in psychiatric medicine there has been a shift over the past century from the use of the notion of 'dangerousness' used in relation to people with psychiatric disorders to that of 'risk'. All insane people were deemed as carrying this potentiality for dangerousness within them, despite their benign exteriors, and were subsequently treated with such preventive strategies as confinement from the rest of society. Risk is therefore more selective and precise, but at the same time applies to a larger group of people than the notion of dangerousness. (cited in Lupton, 1999: 92)

Experts using 'objective facts' calculate risks which are contrasted with the subjective understandings of lay people, but as Lupton reasons, 'such risk calculations tend not to acknowledge the role played by the "ways of seeing" on the part of the experts themselves that produce such calculations. Their understandings of risk are represented as neutral and unbiased' (1999: 19). Reddy questions this and refers to the 'myth of calculability' (1996: 237). Meanwhile Vassilev and Pilgrim argue that:

> psychiatric diagnosis can consequently be accused of being a form of vacuous scientific reification or of simply rubber stamping and codifying decisions made already by others. [Critics have questioned] the expertise of psychiatric diagnosis by invoking 'common sense' and arguing that the average lay person is just as capable at spotting madness as an expert witness. (2007: 349)

The responsibility for risk, in the last resort, has shifted towards professionals of social welfare agencies. Thus social workers, situated between the individual citizen and society, are in the unenviable position of being ascribed the 'risky' role of having to deal with the unpredictabilities, improbabilities and impossibilities of risk – be they categorized as high, medium or low. However, in this world of uncertainties, Fook concludes that uncertainty is not *the* defining characteristic of social work but rather, 'contextuality, or the ability to respond meaningfully in relation to different and changing contexts' (2007: 39).

Reflection exercise

How can social work practice in mental health be effective in responding to 'risky', uncertain situations?

THE POLITICS OF COMPULSORY DETENTION AND TREATMENT

Tensions clearly exist between the government's preoccupation with risk and control and the maintenance of the civil rights and liberty of people in mental distress.

Social work by its very nature often finds itself in the middle of such tension. As a result, as Webb points out:

> Social work in the last 15 years, damaged by successive child abuse scandals has embraced the language of risk and accountability much as have other public institutions. Targets, performance measures and lists of procedures issuing from central government have offered a 'calculative technology' for the assessment and constraining of risky situations. Of course the further burdening of already over-worked social care personnel leads to the opening up of more risk. (2006: 3)

Current techniques, methods and the apparatus of social work; systems and processes (technologies of care), 'including procedural guidelines, case reporting systems, care management, information and data banks are mobilized to shore up the fragile professional status of social work' (2006: 142). Webb argues that the new 'technologies of care' are implicated in the deskilling of social work practice – 'care management, for example, tends to be overly preoccupied with the assessment of need and risk and the matching of available services for service users, rather than relationship building or therapeutic direct work' (2006: 143).

With reference to Grounds (1996), Kemshall argues that disquiet about the management of the mentally distressed in the community was fuelled by a new generation of inquiry reports from the late 1980s onwards: 'The cumulative impact of the inquiry recommendations and attendant publicity subtly moved the mental health agenda from treatment and rehabilitation to control and surveillance. Risk and protection began to dominate the mental health policy agenda' (2002: 98). While the asylums have disappeared, secure containment of the mentally distressed has been achieved with the increased use of compulsory detention, as government policy focuses on the protection of the public. As McLaughlin wryly comments, 'if we dismiss the possibility that the long sought but elusive "schizophrenia gene" has infiltrated the water supply, we have to look for social not medical processes to explain the rapid rise in compulsory admissions in the past decade' (2008: 96). The rights of patients, despite government rhetoric, now take second place to the possible risks they may present. 'Assertive outreach' is to be used for those who are resistant to services (Kemshall, 2002), supported by the use of what Newnes and Holmes describe as 'coercive psychiatry' (1999: 276).

The introduction of the controversial SCT and CTO in the MHA 2007 follows a similar theme, adding a further mechanism of control for those in mental distress. The somewhat minimalist public perception, peddled by the media, is that people in mental distress commit violent acts because they will not take their medication, so it follows that the authorities must make them. However, the following points need to be weighed against the arguments for the CTO:

- Drugs do not cure mental illness as insulin remedies diabetes (Rogers and Pilgrim, 2001: 220).
- Medication given for mental disorder can have adverse side effects (McLaughlin, 2008: 91).
- There is conflict between the HRA 1998 and the MHA 1983 regarding citizens' rights.
- Many professionals see the actual process as unworkable.

- It is counter productive as it introduces fear and mistrust into a therapeutic relationship and could lead to many people being reluctant to seek the care they need.
- Those in mental distress can just 'go missing'.
- Alcohol and substance misuse adversely affect drugs.
- Many psychiatrists are hostile to the CTO because it will extend the use of compulsory powers to a wider group of patients, put more pressure on services and it infringes human rights.

Vassilev and Pilgrim argue that 'the regulation of mental disorder is increasingly dominated by formal rules originating from the political and legal systems'. Using the notions of 'risk' and 'trust' they are led to the conclusion 'that "mental health services" are a myth'. They further argue:

> If taken literally, we would expect 'mental health services' to be about 'mental health' and that they would be 'services'. Clearly they are not about promoting mental health or even ensuring mental health gain. There are simply too many iatrogenic risks and consequences entailed in becoming a psychiatric patient to justify any notion of mental health improvement. (2007: 355)

In short, they are not mental health services but mental health controls.

THE HUMAN RIGHTS ACT 1998

> ### Reflection exercise
>
> What do you understand by the term 'human rights'? How does the law deal with competing rights claims?

The roots of human rights legislation were established following the atrocities committed during the Second World War. To avoid the reoccurrence of such acts countries joined together to form the United Nations. In 1948 the United Nations published the *Universal Declaration of Human Rights* containing 30 articles. These were embedded and extended in the Convention for the Protection of Human Rights and Fundamental Freedoms (also known as the European Convention on Human Rights) published by the Council of Europe in 1950. The European Convention on Human Rights was incorporated into UK law in the shape of the Human Rights Act 1998. The European Court of Human Rights was established in 1959 in Strasbourg and since 1966 a European citizen could petition the court for a violation of one or more of its Articles. However, the petition needed to demonstrate that all domestic remedies had been exhausted before being heard by the European Court which had the disadvantages of being expensive and being subject to long time delays – measured in years. Thus, as Brammer argues, the incorporation of the Convention into UK law was 'partly practical' with the emphasis in the HRA 1998 on 'bringing rights home' (2007: 125). It remains the case, however, that the European Court of Human Rights may still be approached when all other avenues for redress in the UK are exhausted.

Most, but not all, of the articles in the European Convention on Human Rights are incorporated into the HRA 1998 including:

- the right to life
- freedom from torture and degraded treatment
- freedom from slavery and forced labour
- the right to liberty
- the right to a fair trial
- the right not to be punished for something that wasn't a crime when you did it
- the right to respect for private and family life
- freedom of thought, conscience and religion
- freedom of expression
- freedom of assembly and association
- the right to marry or form a civil partnership and start a family
- the right not to be discriminated against in respect of these rights and freedoms
- the right to own property
- the right to an education
- the right to participate in free elections.

Rights are divided into three categories namely:

- *Absolute rights* – those which cannot be restricted in any circumstances and violation claims are not balanced against any general public interest (for example, freedom from torture, inhuman and degrading treatment; freedom from slavery).
- *Limited rights* – where a right is established but there are some limitations (for example, right to liberty, right to life).
- *Qualified rights* – where rights are set but can be interfered with under certain circumstances (for example, right to respect for private and family life, freedom of expression, and freedom of thought, conscience and religion).

It can be seen that many of the articles have the potential to connect with and question social work practice in the area of mental health, especially around issues of compulsory detention and forced medication. The HRA 1998 dictates that public bodies must respect Convention rights in all that they do. Nevertheless, it has to be borne in mind that human rights legislation is not a panacea for all ills. A decade after its inception, the impact of the HRA 1998 has been reviewed by a number of agencies, such as the British Institute of Human Rights (2002) and the Audit Commission (2003). Recently the government commissioned the Human Rights Insight Project to provide an evidence base for human rights policy development 'after a number of independent reports by expert bodies concluded that the potential of the HRA to improve the lives of people in this country was not yet being realised' (Ministry of Justice, 2008: ii). The Project report cites the conclusions of The Parliamentary Joint Committee on Human Rights in 2003:

> The Act has not given birth to a culture of respect for human rights or made human rights a core activity of public authorities ... Too often human rights are looked upon as something from which the state needs to defend itself, rather than to promote as its core ethical values. There is a failure to recognize the part that they could play in promoting social justice and social inclusion and in the drive to improve public services. We have found widespread evidence of a lack of respect for the rights of those who use public services, especially the rights of those who are most vulnerable and in need of protection. (Ministry of Justice, 2008: iii)

The issue of human rights plays an important role in the area of mental health. Decisions about a person's liberty; their right to determine their own future when in mental distress and not to be subject to the omnipotent power of the state are, as Johns argues, 'not just legal issues ... they are fundamental debates about values and ethics in social work' (2007: 4).

THE CENTRALITY OF VALUES AND ETHICS TO SOCIAL WORK PRACTICE IN MENTAL HEALTH

Social workers are positioned somewhat uncomfortably at the interface between individuals, families or communities and the all powerful state. While the great majority of prospective social work students say at interview that they want to enter the profession to 'help people' (and that certainly reflects how the profession is 'marketed' in contemporary recruitment advertisements), the stark reality is that social work is an activity that is inherently controversial by virtue of the statutory authority invested in social workers to intervene in the lives of citizens, whether or not they want such intervention. Social workers are expected to manage competing and often contradictory demands in the face of, at best, public suspicion and, at worst, outright antagonism (as witnessed in relentless vilification from the tabloid media). Clearly it is vital in a context such as this that social work students develop a sound understanding of the significance of the way in which values and ethics underpin social work practice.

Reflection exercise: exploring your own values

'Social worker students need to explore and clarify their own values before they are faced with these challenges. A well-developed value base – and an ability to reflect on value questions – is a necessary tool for a confident and competent practitioner' (Beckett and Maynard, 2005: 1).

What personal values are important to you? Where do you think these values come from? How do you think these values have influenced your decision to enter social work?

When a person undertakes professional social work training, 'values' necessarily move beyond the personal and they are expected to consider competing values and value systems to their own when making judgements and decisions. First, all social workers are bound by the General Social Care Council *Codes of Practice* (GSCC, 2002) which sets out respective responsibilities for social care workers and employers. Second, values (more often expressed as 'principles') are evident (whether implicitly or explicitly) in all official government policies, legislation and associated guidance. Third, social workers will be expected to adhere to the values expressed in the policy statements produced by their individual employing social work agency. There are many additional frameworks and guidelines that social workers are expected to consult, some of which are generic in their focus, such as the GSCC (2008) *Roles and Tasks of Social Workers* and the BASW (2002) *Code of Ethics for Social Work* while others are specific to particular contexts of practice, such as the National Framework of Values for Mental Health (DH, 2004, Appendix B) included below.

The National Framework of Values for Mental Health

The work of the National Institute for Mental Health in England (NIMHE) on values in mental health care is guided by three principles of values-based practice:

1) **Recognition** – NIMHE recognises the role of values alongside evidence in all areas of mental health policy and practice.
2) **Raising Awareness** – NIMHE is committed to raising awareness of the values involved in different contexts, the role/s they play and their impact on practice in mental health.
3) **Respect** – NIMHE respects diversity of values and will support ways of working with such diversity that makes the principle of service-user centrality a unifying focus for practice. This means that the values of each individual service user/client and their communities must be the starting point and key determinant for all actions by professionals.

Respect for diversity of values encompasses a number of specific policies and principles concerned with equality of citizenship. In particular, it is anti-discriminatory because discrimination in all its forms is intolerant of diversity. Thus respect for diversity of values has the consequence that it is unacceptable (and unlawful in some instances) to discriminate on grounds such as gender, sexual orientation, class, age, abilities, religion, race, culture or language.

Respect for diversity within mental health is also:

- *user-centred* – it puts respect for the values of individual users at the centre of policy and practice;

(Continued)

- *recovery oriented* – it recognises that building on the personal strengths and resiliencies of individual users, and on their cultural and racial characteristics, there are many diverse routes to recovery;
- *multidisciplinary* – it requires that respect be reciprocal, at a personal level (between service users, their family members, friends, communities and providers), between different provider disciplines (such as nursing, psychology, psychiatry, occupational therapy, medicine, social work), and between different organisations (including health, social care, local authority housing, voluntary organisations, community groups, faith communities and other social support services);
- *dynamic* – it is open and responsive to change;
- *reflective* – it combines self monitoring and self management with positive self regard;
- *balanced* – it emphasises positive as well as negative values;
- *relational* – it puts positive working relationships supported by good communication skills at the heart of practice.

NIMHE will encourage educational and research initiatives aimed at developing the capabilities (the awareness, attitudes, knowledge and skills) needed to deliver mental health services that will give effect to the principles of values-based practice.

(DH, 2004: Appendix B)

While articulating what ought to happen is relatively easy, as discussed earlier in this chapter, it is once social workers are required to put such values into action that they often experience considerable tension and contradiction in their role. Reconciling conflicts between personal values and limited options in the real world of decision-making is intensely demanding and stressful. Taking control and autonomy away from an individual in mental distress in order to protect that person and, very rarely, others is a situation that inevitably poses one of the most difficult ethical challenges to those practitioners committed to the core values of personal autonomy, freedom of choice and an anti-oppressive approach. The role of the social worker in these situations is demanding and difficult. S/he will be expected to weigh up and resolve competing principles and values. Each position will have strengths and weaknesses and it is the social worker's job to balance these in order to arrive at a decision.

CHAPTER SUMMARY

A good knowledge of legislation is central to good social work practice. Legislation is dynamic, often modified by case law and governmental policy. Rights and responsibilities mix with moral and ethical positions and cause tensions between professionals working in the area as well as service users and their carers. Achieving the 'risk balance' between the protection of the public and the protection of the individual is often very difficult. Thus social workers find themselves caught between the power of the state and the protection of those in mental distress. In a liberal democratic society where the sanctity of freedom is revered, involvement in a system that can take away an individual's liberty requires the utmost sensitivity and care.

Further reading/resources

The Mental Health Act 1983. London: HMSO.
The Mental Health Act 2007. London: HMSO.
Department of Health (DH) (2008) *Reference Guide to the Mental Health Act 1983*. London: TSO.
Department of Health (DH) (2008) *Code of Practice: Mental Health Act 1983* (revised May 2008). London: TSO.
www.equalityhumanrights.com – Equality and Human Rights Commission.
www.mind.org.uk – National Association for Mental Health.
www.yourrights.org.uk – Liberty.

5 WHAT WORKS IN PROMOTING RECOVERY?

Evidence-based practice and the dynamics of power in mental health research

This chapter can be used to support the development of knowledge and skills in professional social work as follows:

National Occupational Standards for Social Work

Key Role 1: Prepare for and work with individuals, families, carers, groups and communities to assess their needs and circumstances

- Prepare for social work contact and involvement
- Work with individuals, families, carers, groups and communities to help them make informed decisions
- Assess needs and options to recommend a course of action.

Key Role 2: Plan, carry out, review and evaluate social work practice, with individuals, families, carers, groups and communities and other professionals

- Prepare, produce, implement and evaluate plans with individuals, families, carers, groups, communities and professional colleagues
- Address behaviour which presents a risk to individuals, families, carers, groups, communities.

Key Role 6: Demonstrate professional competence in social work practice

- Research, analyse, evaluate, and use current knowledge of best social work practice
- Work within agreed standards of social work practice and ensure own professional development
- Managing complex ethical issues, dilemmas and conflicts
- Contribute to the promotion of best social work practice.

(TOPPS England, 2002)

Academic Standards for Social Work

Honours graduates in social work:

5.1 should acquire, critically evaluate, apply and integrate knowledge and understanding in relation to:

5.1.1 Social work services, service users and carers

- the social processes (associated with, for example, poverty, migration, unemployment, poor health, disablement, lack of education and other sources of disadvantage) that lead to marginalisation, isolation and exclusion and their impact on the demand for social work services
- explanations of the links between definitional processes contributing to social differences (for example, social class, gender, ethnic differences, age, sexuality and religious belief) to the problems of inequality and differential need faced by service users
- the nature and validity of different definitions of, and explanations for, the characteristics and circumstances of service users and the services required by them, drawing on knowledge from research, practice experience, and from service users and carers.

5.1.4 Social work theory

- research-based concepts and critical explanations from social work theory and other disciplines that contribute to the knowledge base of social work, including their distinctive epistemological status and application to practice
- the relevance of sociological perspectives to understanding societal and structural influences on human behaviour at individual, group and community levels
- the relevance of psychological and physiological perspectives to understanding individual and social development and functioning.

5.5.3 should be able to analyse and synthesise information gathered for problem solving purposes to:

- assess the merits of contrasting theories, explanations, research, policies and procedures
- critically analyse and take account of the impact of inequality and discrimination in work with people in particular contexts and problem situations.

(QAA, 2008)

Key themes in this chapter

- Mental health treatment as a contested arena
- Biological approaches to managing mental distress

(Continued)

- Psychological approaches to managing mental distress
- Social approaches to managing mental distress
- The recovery agenda in mental health care
- Evidence-based practice – what counts as evidence and who decides?

INTRODUCTION

This chapter introduces some of the current approaches to managing mental distress and promoting recovery. Given the tensions and contradictions surrounding the different concepts and theories used to describe and understand mental health and mental distress, it is vital that practitioners also appreciate the equally diverse, often antagonistic, nature of the treatment approaches that have evolved in this field over time. We begin with a historical discussion of the contested nature of mental health treatments before going on to outline and evaluate some of the main contemporary approaches to treating mental distress (physical, psychological and social). The discussion moves on to focus on recent developments around the notion of 'recovery' in mental health care, emphasizing the importance of user-defined notions of what 'recovery' means and how best to promote it. Recognizing the importance of incorporating up to date research into professional mental health practice, we then engage in a critical analysis of the evidence-based practice (EBP) approach to mental health research and evaluation. The discussion concludes by acknowledging that those in mental distress and their carers are 'experts by experience' and asserts the centrality and validity of user-focused and user-led approaches to research and evaluation.

MENTAL HEALTH TREATMENT AS A CONTESTED ARENA

Having established in Chapter 1 that the boundaries around what constitutes mental distress are uncertain and heavily disputed, it should come as no surprise to learn that the same is true regarding approaches to understanding what works in the treatment of mental distress. The historical development of treatment approaches in mental health practice is closely associated with changing understandings of the nature of mental distress and with the emergence of psychiatry both as a body of knowledge and a profession that has primary clinical and legal responsibility for the management of the mentally distressed. From the earliest days of psychiatric practice approaches to treating and managing the mentally distressed were contested and controversial since they were primarily concerned with forced incarceration and crude physical and chemical attempts to calm or restrain individuals. Almost inevitably then, psychiatry became associated with coercive control – a negative legacy that persists to this day. For many critical commentators it is the blurring of treatment and control functions in mental health practice that creates an intrinsically antagonistic relationship between psychiatry and the mentally distressed (Fennell, 1996).

Currently, all patients (other than those who are legally compelled under the Mental Health Act 1983) have a right to refuse psychiatric treatment or must give legally valid consent to receiving it. This consent must be obtained without undue pressure of any kind and patients must also be given full information on the nature and purpose of the treatment, including any side effects. Unfortunately there is evidence to suggest that these conditions are not always met (Cobb, 1993; Rogers et al., 1993). Furthermore, as already discussed in Chapter 4, while only a minority of users are subject to the provisions of the Mental Health Act 1983, it is the ever-present threat of compulsory detention and treatment without consent that makes for a tense and difficult relationship between the mentally distressed and mental health professionals. This harsh reality must be borne in mind throughout the following discussion of approaches to managing mental distress.

BIOLOGICAL APPROACHES TO MANAGING MENTAL DISTRESS

The medical model of mental health promotes the idea that mental health problems are akin to physical illness conditions and are therefore amenable to technological solutions, particularly through biological treatments. Biological treatments have a long and controversial history in psychiatry. Their development in the eighteenth, nineteenth and early twentieth centuries reflected the emergence and consolidation of a medical monopoly over the care and treatment of the mentally distressed. While some of the more 'exotic' approaches to psychiatric treatment have long since been discarded, (such as revolving chairs; bleeding, purging and vomiting; water therapy and insulin coma therapy) the majority of people who use mental health services continue to be treated with interventions directed at the human body, more specifically, the brain.

Electroconvulsive Therapy (ECT)

Electroconvulsive Therapy was first introduced into psychiatric practice in Britain in 1938 based on the research findings of two Italian psychiatrists, Cerletti and Bini who demonstrated that shock-induced convulsions were apparently effective in treating severe mental illness. The UK National Institute for Health and Clinical Excellence (NICE) describes the procedure as follows:

> During ECT, an electrical current is passed briefly through the brain, via electrodes applied to the scalp, to induce generalised seizure activity. The individual receiving treatment is placed under general anaesthetic and muscle relaxants are given to prevent body spasms. (NICE, 2003: 9)

NICE acknowledges that there is no clear evidence regarding how ECT works and 'no conclusive evidence to support [its] effectiveness ... beyond the short term or that it is more beneficial as a maintenance therapy in depressive illness than currently available pharmacological alternatives' (2003: 16). Nevertheless, it recommends ECT for the treatment of severe depressive illness, a prolonged or severe manic episode or catatonia 'to achieve rapid and short-term improvement of an individual's severe symptoms after an adequate trial of other treatment options has proven ineffective and/or when the situation is considered to be potentially life-threatening' (2003: 20).

Always a controversial treatment, ECT often arouses strong ethical objections, in part due to its symbolic associations with acts of torture, control and electrocution. Its legitimacy was particularly challenged when the subject was brought to a mass audience via the film version of Ken Kesey's *One Flew Over the Cuckoo's Nest* in 1975. Although administrations of ECT have declined significantly since then, many practitioners continue to advocate its use. According to the UK Department of Health (DH, 2003b), 12,800 ECT treatments were administered to 2,272 people in England in 2002, however, concern has been expressed about serious under-reporting. The Mental Health Act Commission (MHAC, 2004) found that 10 per cent of facilities providing ECT could not provide a register of this treatment.

Critics suggest that there is very little evidence that ECT is helpful and a good deal of evidence that it can be very harmful (Ruthen, 2006). Breggin (2008) is one of the fiercest critics of the continued use of ECT arguing that it damages the brain. He explains that ECT produces the same acute confusional state that occurs after any trauma to the brain – as for example through epilepsy, strangulation, suffocation or a blow to the head. However, while this acute reaction usually subsides in a few hours other more serious effects may not – most notably short- and long-term memory loss and impaired mental functioning, as in the case of Pat Butterfield, founder of the user support group ECT Anonymous:

> It robbed me of my memories. I only knew who my friends were because they kept coming in to see me. I lost all my confidence because I couldn't remember how to do things. I still have problems dealing with a lot of information. I used to be a multi-tasker, but I have problems even sorting things out in sequence now. I am also terrified of hospitals and doctors. I have never been back to one, I have never even been to see my GP since. I certainly did not give my informed consent to the procedure that I underwent. No one told me what the side effects could be. No one even explained to me what would happen. I have never been able to go back to work, and I certainly wouldn't have got as far as I have without the help of my family and friends. (*BBC News*, 26 January 2000)

A Mental Health Foundation study (Faulkner, 1997) found that of the 27 per cent of patients who had received ECT, 30 per cent found it helpful or helpful at times and 47 per cent had found it unhelpful. Research by Johnstone (1999) suggests that the patient's experience of ECT is characterized by powerlessness, control and conformity and therefore may exacerbate psychological problems rather than alleviate them. She also argues that ECT may undermine the relationship between mental health professionals and patients and, therefore, may impede the therapeutic process. There are also particular concerns that ECT is used disproportionately among older women – 1,600 female patients received the treatment in 2002 as compared with 700 male patients (DH, 2003b).

Drug Treatments

Since the mid-1950s, psychiatry's frontline response to mental distress has been psychoactive drugs. The great majority of psychiatric research is currently dominated by a focus on neurotransmitter function, positing the theory of bio-chemical imbalances in the brain which can be 'corrected' with appropriate drug treatments. Most drugs used in the treatment of mental distress fall into four main categories: anti-anxiety drugs; anti-depressants; anti-psychotics; and mood stabilizers. Western society is consuming increasing quantities of psychoactive medication. For example, in the UK the use of anti-depressant medication increased by 234 per cent in the 10 years up to 2002 (NICE, 2004, cited in Moncrieff, 2006). The number of prescriptions for anti-depressants hit a record high of more than 31 million in England in 2006. In the USA 11 per cent of women and 5 per cent of men now take anti-depressants (Stagnitti, 2005, cited in Moncrieff, 2006). Prozac alone is taken by more than 40 million people worldwide. However, there is mounting evidence pointing to the limited effectiveness and potentially harmful effects of drug treatments such as these. Prescriptions for Selective Serotonin Reuptake Inhibitors (SSRIs), which include drugs such as Seroxat and Prozac, rose by 10 per cent in England in 2006 from 14.7m to 16.2m even though guidance from NICE in 2004 stated that they should not be a first choice treatment for mild to moderate depression because of longstanding concerns that these drugs are linked to suicidal thoughts and self-harm in some cases.

Researchers from the University of Hull (Kirsch et al., 2008) conducted a meta-analysis of research data obtained from 47 clinical trials reporting on the effectiveness of anti-depressant medication. According to lead researcher Professor Irving Kirsch 'the difference in improvement between patients taking placebos and patients taking anti-depressants is not very great. This means that depressed people can improve without chemical treatments' (Kirsch, *BBC News*, 26 February 2008). He concluded, 'given these results, there seems little reason to prescribe anti-depressant medication to any but the most severely depressed patients, unless alternative treatments have failed to provide a benefit'.

Many other psychiatric drug treatments have been found to produce 'iatrogenic' effects – that is a tendency to produce new forms of sickness in those they aim to treat. For example, research studies have generally concluded that anti-psychotic drugs are effective in helping to control the acute symptoms associated with severe mental illness and may also help to maintain social functioning if taken regularly. However, for many people any potential benefits are counterbalanced by severe side effects. Acute movement disorders that resemble Parkinson's disease may appear soon after commencing treatment. These include a general slowing down in movement and responsiveness to the environment, along with tremor, writhing movements and a 'zombie-like' expression. Drug-induced agitation and depression may also follow – a condition known as *akathesia* – characterized by a severe restlessness and inability to keep still. The most disabling long-term side effect is *tardive dyskinesia* – a neurological disorder that may emerge after years of prolonged exposure to anti-psychotic medication. This disorder is characterized by involuntary movements of the jaw, tongue, lips and face which may not become apparent until the medication is reduced or stopped. These side effects are extremely difficult to treat once established and are generally irreversible (Breggin, 2008; Thomas, 1997). Furthermore, the bizarre uncontrollable mannerisms induced by anti-psychotic medication are intensely stigmatizing. Concern has also been expressed that high doses of powerful anti-psychotic medication are often prescribed in dangerous combinations with a significant risk of sudden death. Even more worrying is their disproportionate and/or inappropriate use as a management tool for particular groups of people, such as older people, the learning disabled, prisoners and African-Caribbean men (MIND, 2001a).

Reflection exercise

Why do you think drug treatments dominate mental health care? What are the implications of this?

The Persistence of Medical Hegemony in Mental Health Care

Despite substantial investment in bio-medically driven research, it remains the case that the great bulk of what psychiatrists call 'mental illness' actually has no proven physical cause. Drug treatments may be used to relieve some of the 'symptoms' or manifestations of mental distress, but this does not imply that they 'cure' anything. As Tew points out:

> there is so far little evidence that a primary reliance on biomedical strategies for working with people with mental distress has been successful in terms of promoting longer term recovery [indeed] rates of recovery from schizophrenia (defined in terms of remission of symptomatology) have not improved significantly over the last fifty years. (2002: 143)

Nevertheless, due to the power of medical hegemony in this field, there remains a misplaced assumption that science has proven the case, to the detriment of users of mental health services. Dr Bruce G. Charlton from the Department of Anatomy at the University of Glasgow has criticized biological psychiatry for its reductionism, arguing:

> the implicit rationale or philosophy underlying much biological psychiatric research [is] the idea that psychiatric illness is caused by alterations in neurotransmitter function. This view

is so firmly embedded in most research programmes that ... we forget that there is in fact no direct evidence to link any specific psychiatric diagnosis with a neurotransmitter change. (cited in Marshall, 1996)

There is obviously a need for a balanced approach to understanding the role of physical treatments for mental distress, recognizing that medication has a potentially useful but nonetheless limited role as one aspect of the help that those in mental distress might choose to receive. However, it is also evident that the mental health system is extremely resistant to change. According to Rogers and Pilgrim 'whilst 98 per cent of British psychiatric patients receive drug treatment, only 60 per cent report receiving some form of psychological intervention, and some of this is obtained outside the NHS' (2003: 208). Drug treatments are relatively quick and easy to administer when compared with psychological interventions so it is perhaps unsurprising that busy GPs and psychiatrists rely so heavily on them. Significantly, however, research by the University of Essex commissioned by MIND (2007b) reports that 93 per cent of GPs have prescribed drugs due to lack of any real alternatives. Understandably, users of mental health services and advocacy groups have been critical of the over-reliance on drugs and have demanded greater access to psychological therapies (Mental Health Foundation, MIND, Rethink, Sainsbury Centre for Mental Health and Young Minds, 2006).

PSYCHOLOGICAL APPROACHES TO MANAGING MENTAL DISTRESS

Historically, psychological therapies have always represented a potential challenge to the dominance of medical psychiatry in understanding and 'treating' mental distress; whether practised by those who were medical doctors (as for example with Sigmund Freud, Pierre Janet, Alfred Adler and Carl Jung) or non-physicians (such as B.F. Skinner, Aaron Beck and Carl Rogers) (Coppock and Hopton, 2000). However, such is the power of medical hegemony in psychiatry that 'talking therapies' have long existed in the shadow of the medical model.

A wide range of activities are encompassed in the term 'therapy', from brief supportive discussions with someone with little or no specialist training, to intensive work with a highly trained practitioner over periods of months or years. However, most practitioners will usually be trained in one or more of the orthodox therapies – psychodynamic therapy; cognitive/behaviour therapy; or person-centred therapy. Each of these is briefly outlined below.

Psychodynamic Therapy

This model originates in the work of Sigmund Freud in the late nineteenth century and has been revised and developed by other significant twentieth century theorists such as Anna Freud, Melanie Klein and Erik Erikson. In very basic terms, psychodynamic theory focuses on the ways in which past experiences (especially early childhood experiences) and emotions, repressed in the unconscious, may influence thoughts, feelings and behaviours in the present. It is believed that significant relationships and traumas may be replayed with other people later in life, causing personal 'dysfunction' or 'dysfunctional' interpersonal relationships. The psychodynamic therapist explores these experiences and emotions with the client, aiming to provide a 'blank screen' onto which the client 'transfers' feelings about these significant relationships. The therapist facilitates the development of the client's 'insight' into how s/he behaves in relationships with others so that s/he can understand and change responses that are causing problems.

Cognitive/behaviour Therapy

During the 1970s and 1980s behaviour therapy (also known as behaviour modification) was very much in vogue in mental health services. Based on the work of B.F. Skinner, behavioural therapy is based on the theory that patterns of behaviour, such as phobic reactions, obsessions and severe anxiety, are learned behaviours which can be eradicated and replaced with more constructive behaviours. Therapists seek to control clients' environments and manipulate the consequences of their behaviours in order to eliminate some and encourage others. The ethics of this approach were increasingly called into question and it has now been largely displaced by cognitive behaviour therapy (CBT). Cognitive behaviour therapy emanates from the work of Aaron Beck and Albert Ellis in the 1960s and 1970s and was originally developed as a treatment for people diagnosed with depression. It has since been used in the treatment of a much wider range of diagnosed conditions. The central theoretical argument is that it is a person's perception of events rather than the events themselves that determines their behaviour. Cognitive therapists suggest that psychological distress is caused by distorted thoughts about events giving rise to distressed emotions. They aim to teach the client new skills in managing their mental distress by helping them to become aware of the thought distortions which are causing the distress, and of behavioural patterns which are reinforcing it, and to correct them. The CBT approach usually focuses on difficulties in the here and now, and relies on the therapist and user developing a shared view of the individual's problem. This then leads to identification of personalized, usually time-limited, therapy goals and strategies which are continually monitored and evaluated. CBT practitioners claim that this approach is inherently empowering in nature, since the outcome focuses on specific psychological and practical skills (for example in reflecting on and exploring the meaning attributed to events and situations and re-evaluation of those meanings) aimed at enabling the client to tackle their problems by harnessing their own resources. The acquisition and utilization of such skills is seen as the main goal, and the active component in promoting change with an emphasis on putting what has been learned into practice between sessions through 'homework'.

Person-centred Therapy

The most widely practised school of therapy in counselling contexts is person-centred therapy. This is based on the work of the American psychologist Carl Rogers who popularized the approach in the 1950s. Rogers argued that human beings need to realize their full intellectual, emotional and creative potential. However, this process requires favourable conditions – unconditional acceptance and positive regard by others – otherwise dissonance will occur between the person's image of themselves and the image reflected back to them by others. When a person becomes overly dependent on other people's perceptions this results in a weak and fragmented sense of self. Person-centred therapy is based on three core conditions – 'unconditional positive regard', 'empathic understanding' and 'congruence'. The therapist enables the client to develop and grow in their own way; to strengthen and expand their own identity and to become the person that they 'really' are, independent of the pressures of others to act or think in particular ways. Person-centred therapy sessions usually involve the client doing most of the talking whilst the therapist's responses focus on conveying an empathic understanding of the client's world. The therapist's role is that of a non-directive facilitator, encouraging the client to explore their inner world in order to enhance their own ability to resolve their problems.

Talking Therapies – a Risk Free Alternative to Medication?

According to NICE (2007a, 2007b) psychological therapies are just as effective as drug treatments when treating anxiety and depression. However, such therapies are in very short supply. For example, the average waiting list for CBT in the UK is 18 months; although the UK Government has recently committed itself to substantially improving access to psychological therapies by 2010 (*BBC News*, 11 October 2007). Nevertheless, despite the high demand for psychological therapies, there are those who are sceptical, particularly regarding the extent to which they offer a genuine alternative to drug treatments. While there is evidence to suggest that CBT and other therapies can be highly effective, they should not be seen as a quick solution and are not a panacea for everyone:

> CBT is the new black in mental health. The trouble is that it works mainly for people with mild to moderate depression. It rarely works for people with more severe forms of depression or anxiety ... GPs, pressed for time and under pressure from directives, may be tempted to prescribe CBT as a cure for all distress which is quite wrong ... (contributor, *PM Programme Blog*, BBC Radio 4, 10 October 2007)

Many of the reservations expressed by users relate to the potential for therapists to control or dominate them:

> I had ten months of CBT at my local surgery and believe me it all depends on what you believe and your personal experience. The therapist was basically a good person but

tried in vain to brainwash me into believing things were not as bad as I saw them. The therapy seemed useless in doing anything about the personal sense of injustice I had because of my experience and rejection at the hands of others. In the end it became an exercise in being led to believe that if I didn't agree with the therapist, then I didn't want to get better. (contributor, *PM Programme Blog*, BBC Radio 4, 10 October 2007)

Some research studies have revealed serious emotional, physical and sexual abuse of clients by therapists (Masson, 1990; Rutter, 1995; Wood, 1993). Additionally, it is evident that psychological therapies are as open to charges of inherent bias and stereotyping in relation to class, race, gender, sexuality and age as any other mental health intervention (Wood, 1993).

> **Reflection exercise**
>
> What are the advantages and disadvantages of talking therapies?

SOCIAL APPROACHES TO MANAGING MENTAL DISTRESS

> As human beings our thoughts, our emotions and our behaviours are always related to the context of our lives. How we see ourselves, the words we use to describe our experiences, our concerns and our priorities are all bound up with the social world in which we live. Contrary to the ideology of biological psychiatry, the lived experience of human beings will never be explained by way of reference to the make-up of the brain alone. (Bracken, 2002: 26)

The quotation above challenges us to look beyond the scope of medical or psychological interventions in mental health care towards the social and environmental contexts of the lives of the mentally distressed. As one user has commented, 'CBT on its own won't do an individual much good if part of the problem lies in the way that they live, their housing or working conditions' (Contributor, *PM Programme Blog*, BBC Radio 4, 10 October 2007).

The social model of mental distress was popularized with the publication of the ground-breaking study, *Social Origins of Depression* by Brown and Harris in 1978. These researchers found a prevalence rate of depression in working-class women three times that of their middle-class group. As well as class differences they also found a clear association of depression with what they termed 'vulnerability factors' such as having three or more children under 14 years old living at home, lack of an intimate confiding relationship, lack of either full-time or part-time employment and having lost a mother before the age of 11 years.

Contemporary advocates of the social model point out that 'over and above any biological predisposing factors, evidence suggests that a variety of social factors may play a major role in contributing to longer term vulnerability to breakdown or distress' (Tew, 2002: 148). There is evidence to suggest that policies and services that are targeted at reducing the impact of profound inequalities in society and their consequences in the form of unemployment, poor housing, poverty, stigma and social isolation have a more positive impact on recovery rates (WHO, 2004). In the UK, the Department of Health acknowledges that mental health problems can result from the range of adverse factors associated with social exclusion and can also be a cause of social exclusion. To that end, Standard 1 of the *National Service Framework for Mental Health* states that 'health and social services should promote mental health for all, working with individuals and communities and combat discrimination against individuals and groups with mental health problems, and promote their social inclusion' (DH, 1999a: 14). However, this cannot be achieved without recourse to a social model of mental distress that informs interventions targeted at the root causes of poor mental health.

Central to the social model is the proposition that mental distress may be understood as a meaningful response to problematic life experiences – in particular experiences of oppression, exclusion and powerlessness. Therefore, rather than constituting 'illnesses' as such, 'behaviours defined as symptoms and disorders are best understood as creative responses to difficult personal and social histories, rooted in a person's experience of oppression(s)' (Williams, 1999: 31). This implies the need for a professional response that involves supporting individuals on their journey towards recovery and challenging structural inequalities that give rise to their mental distress, such as poverty, racism, sexism, ageism and homophobia. As Tew points out:

> Where this approach differs so markedly from the medical model is that what would have been seen just as clusters of 'symptoms' come alive as meaningful responses to sequences of often horrendous life circumstances. This sets the foundations for new forms of alliance and dialogue between social worker and user, one that starts with a validation of the user's immense expertise in living with and surviving situations that may be well beyond the direct experience of the worker. (2002: 149)

THE RECOVERY AGENDA IN MENTAL HEALTH CARE

McKnight (1995) argues that there are four central assumptions that characterize the traditional attitude and behaviour of health and social care professionals. These are:

1. The service user is the problem, the professional is the answer.
2. The professional 'remedy' or service defines the need.
3. The 'problem' and the 'solution' are coded into incomprehensible jargon.
4. Professionals decide what 'help' is effective.

These needs-oriented assumptions can disable and disempower the people with whom health and social care professionals come into contact. For McKnight the alternative is to develop policies and activities that recognize and enable the development of people's capacities, skills and assets.

In recent years users of mental health services and mental health professionals have come together to promote the idea of 'recovery' (CSIP, RCPsych and SCIE, 2007; SPN, 2007). In 2001, MIND reported the findings of an extensive survey *Roads to Recovery* in which over half of respondents said that they felt recovered or were coping with their mental distress. Respondents had various diagnoses including depression, schizophrenia, bi-polar disorder, post-traumatic stress disorder and personality disorder.

> **Roads to Recovery (MIND, 2001b)**
>
> Key findings:
>
> - 36% of respondents said they felt recovered
> - 21% of respondents said they were coping
> - 65% of those who felt recovered or were coping said talking to family and friends kept them well; 62% said eating well; 56% said working and volunteering; 54% said hobbies and 50% said physical exercise
> - 62% of those who felt recovered or were coping said the main barrier to recovery was the attitude of the general public; 54% said low self esteem; 50% said the benefits trap and low income; 39% said mental health professionals; 37% said lack of choice in treatments; 37% said acts of discrimination and 25% said racism
> - 47% of those who felt recovered or were coping said support from mental health services *first* helped their recovery; 42% said support from family and friends first helped; 42% said psychiatric drugs; 38% said talking treatments; 31% said GP services; 20% said spirituality/religion and 11% said alternative therapies.

The findings from this research counteract the serious lack of positive messages about how people can learn to live with or 'recover' from their mental distress (see also Heyes, 2005; Simpson, 2004). In this context 'recovery' is about people seeing themselves as capable of finding a positive way forward out of their distress rather than as passive recipients of professional interventions. As Tew argues 'recovery cannot be 'done to' people; it cannot be led by 'experts' who claim to know both the destination and the route by which this is to be reached' (2005: 27). Far from simply accepting an illness diagnosis and learning to manage medication, the idea of recovery puts meanings, relationships and values at the heart of mental health care – it is a *process* not an event.

> To some ... recovery is seen as a negative term associated with illness being 'cured'. The medical model looks to return the patient to the not-ill state. But people have mental illness as an experience, not an objective reality. It is woven into the fabric of who and what they are. (Helm, 2003: 53)

> **Reflection exercise**
>
> What does the term 'recovery' mean to you?

The process of recovery may involve users learning to weave their 'illness experiences' into an integrated sense of self, rather than bracketing them off as 'alien' or 'other'. This is exemplified in the activities of the user-led Hearing Voices Network where users learn and develop strategies to take control of the voice hearing experience rather than seeking to eradicate it (Coleman, 1999; Romme and Escher, 1993). User-led networks such as this also offer important opportunities for mutual support and can provide a focus for campaigning activities, challenging oppressive and discriminatory structures or relationships, or reclaiming aspects of ordinary life, such as decent housing and employment opportunities (Tew, 2002).

The recovery agenda brings together themes and issues that should be familiar to social work – enabling the voice of the service user, anti-oppressive practice and a focus on systems, networks and relationships (Tew, 2002). However, many would argue that these essential dimensions of the 'craft' of social work have been significantly undermined in recent years (Duggan et al., 2002; Jones et al., 2004).

> Many of us entered social work – and many still do – out of a commitment to social justice or, at the very least, to bring about positive change in people's lives ... That potential for social change has all but been squeezed out of social work by the drives towards marketisation and managerialism that have characterised the last decade and a half. (Jones et al., 2004)

In this context it is essential that social work engages with, and learns from, the mental health user movements in ways which will allow new partnerships to form and an ethically engaged social work practice to flourish. Duggan, Cooper and Foster's (2002) proposal for a modern social model in mental health represents a positive way forward.

The modern social model in mental health: key characteristics

- It is based on an understanding of complexity of human health and well being.
- It emphasises the interaction of social factors with those of biology and microbiology in the construction of health and disease.
- It addresses the inner and the outer worlds of individuals, groups and communities.

(Continued)

- It embraces the experiences and supports the social networks of people who are vulnerable and frail.
- It understands and works collaboratively within the institutions of civil society to promote the interests of individuals and communities and to critique and challenge when these are detrimental to these interests.
- It emphasises shared knowledge and shared territory with a range of disciplines and with service users and the general public.
- It emphasises empowerment and capacity building at individual and community level and therefore tolerates and celebrates difference.
- It places equal value on the expertise of service users, carers and the general public but will challenge attitudes and practices that are oppressive, judgemental and destructive.
- It operationalises a critical understanding of the nature of power and hierarchy in the creation of health inequalities and social exclusion.
- It is committed to the development of theory and practice and to the critical evaluation of process and outcome.

(Duggan et al., 2002: 19).

EVIDENCE-BASED PRACTICE – WHAT COUNTS AS EVIDENCE AND WHO DECIDES?

The Relationship Between Drug Companies and Psychiatry

The scientific and objective basis of psychopharmacological research has increasingly been called into question. Psychiatry is an important target for pharmaceutical companies who spend vast amounts of money on advertising and hospitality for psychiatrists and provide generous funding for research that promotes a pro-drug approach (Moncrieff, 2003). This relationship raises important ethical questions about the capacity of drug companies to skew the research agenda in favour of a narrow biological approach to the explanation for and treatment of mental distress. For example, recent studies of the effectiveness of drug treatments for depression reveal how drug companies are selective with the evidence they produce and what they release to clinicians, the patient and the public (Kendall, 2006; Kirsch et al., 2008; Turner et al., 2008). Kendall (2006) highlights how drug companies can distort the production of evidence, for example through the selection of trial participants; the selection of outcomes to report and analyse; and the interpretation of the evidence.

Similarly, Turner et al. (2008) report that the effectiveness of anti-depressants may have been exaggerated because the results of unfavourable studies have not been published. These researchers found that the vast majority of clinical trials which revealed negative or questionable results were not published or were published in a way that made them seem positive. As a result, while published data appears to show that 94 per cent of tests had a positive outcome, in fact the US Food and Drug

Administration found just 51 per cent had a positive outcome. Clearly such publication bias threatens to skew professionals' understanding of how effective a drug is for a particular condition:

> Evidence-based medicine is valuable to the extent that the evidence base is complete and unbiased. Selective publication of clinical trials – and the outcomes within those trials – can lead to unrealistic estimates of drug effectiveness and alter the apparent risk–benefit ratio. We cannot determine whether the bias observed resulted from a failure to submit manuscripts on the part of authors and sponsors, from decisions by journal editors and reviewers not to publish, or both. Selective reporting of clinical trial results may have adverse consequences for researchers, study participants, health care professionals, and patients. (Turner et al., 2008: 252)

These findings suggest that we need to examine carefully the process by which knowledge is created and, perhaps more importantly, how certain kinds of knowledge are valued more highly than others. The World Health Organization (2001c) acknowledges that the production and distribution of knowledge is culturally and politically determined and that historical and contemporary biases in mental health research have resulted in a distorted and incomplete understanding of mental health. It follows therefore that all levels of scientific enquiry, from the formulation of research questions through to design, methodology and interpretation of results need to be open to critical scrutiny. Without the incorporation of good quality critical research about mental health into education and training, mental health practitioners' knowledge will be inaccurate and incomplete.

Evidence-Based Practice (EBP)

Few would dispute that users of services should have access to the best possible care and treatment; that practitioners should be accountable for their interventions and that policy makers should be confident in the knowledge of what works best in mental health care. Moreover, there is a broad consensus of opinion that an 'evidence-based practice' approach to mental health research and evaluation is the means by which this is to be achieved. The EBP approach asserts that there are various types of 'evidence' and that these can be graded along a hierarchy where Level I is considered the best possible.

The hierarchy of evidence

Level I – meta-analysis of randomized control trials (RCTs)
Level II – experimental studies
Level III – well-designed, quasi-experimental studies
Level IV – well-designed, non-experimental studies (comparative, correlational, descriptive, case studies)
Level V – case reports, clinical examples.

This hierarchy is influenced by a particular philosophy of science that privileges the positivist tradition of quantitative research design. The mental health practitioner is usually led to search for sources of evidence that rate highly in terms of this hierarchy – for example those research studies included in scientific internet databases such as the Cochrane Library and Evidence-Based Mental Health. This clearly has implications for the status of qualitative research which occupies the lower/bottom levels of the hierarchy and it is more often this type of research design that characterizes user- and carer-centred research studies. These are issues that have been overlooked in the current climate of enthusiasm for EBP, but we explore some of them here through a series of questions:

To what extent is it possible to acquire objective truth/knowledge about what works in mental health care?

This question is concerned with recognizing that *all* research is inherently political, with practitioners/researchers attached to a particular/preferred theoretical and methodological approach. There is still a great deal of reluctance to acknowledge that the process of building evidence in mental health theory and practice is shaped by values and interpretation. Although it is often argued that the EBP approach offers methodological rigour, conveying a sense of certainty and authority, in reality this is often more illusory than is suggested by the evidence. The argument that the approach is a neutral, context-less methodology that can simply be applied whenever and wherever required is unsustainable (see Black 2001; Faulkner and Thomas, 2002; Reynolds and Trinder, 2000).

To what extent can the EBP approach to research and evaluation in mental health do justice to other forms of knowledge, particularly user and carer perspectives?

This question is concerned with recognizing that knowledge is inextricably linked to power, with some forms of knowledge being privileged over others (Foucault, 1977). The evidence-based practice approach currently adopted in most mental health research and evaluation in the UK privileges professional definitions of what constitutes legitimate knowledge. Within this context, there is limited scope for the voices of the mentally distressed and their carers to be heard. The centrality of experience, narrative, individual, qualitative evidence and analysis within user and carer centred research studies are at odds with the dominant, rational, hierarchy of evidence approach of EBP. The persistence of this hierarchy of evidence approach means that as research *evidence* these studies tend to be seen as 'soft', subordinate to 'hard' scientific mental health research and so risk being marginalized. While such power imbalances exist there is a danger that the messages from user- and carer-centred research will not *directly* inform service development and delivery.

To what extent does the EBP approach facilitate a critical appraisal of the world of professional practice?

The subtleties of the way in which the power relationships between service users and carers and professionals are articulated and sustained in the real world of practice are often overlooked in positivistic research and evaluation. Practitioners derive their understandings and approaches to practice from broad theoretical orientations and their professional training. They operate within a range of organizational and legal structures that define people who use mental health services, and which determine the broader construction of mental health policy, law and practice. However, it is rarely acknowledged that these structures are not fixed but are continually contested and negotiated. They are informed by prevailing *social* constructions of mental health and mental distress that practitioners may find difficult to recognize, and so may constitute a hidden agenda in the dynamic of practice. This suggests that there is a need for a research methodology that enables researchers to engage with this domain in order to expose and correct those elements of practice that militate against the realization of a truly anti-oppressive, empowering practice with the mentally distressed.

Who does EBP benefit? Is 'best-evidence' actually put into practice?

Evidence-based practice emerged in the early 1990s in the wider context of a concern with the application of New Public Management principles in health and social care. Therefore many critics of EBP believe that its popularity has more to do with the managerialist drive towards efficiency, effectiveness and evaluation, characterized by 'best value' and 'performance indicators', than a genuine commitment to best practice. In this sense, where the main focus of concern is the effective management of systems and organizations, EBP may actually be antagonistic to the priorities of users and carers. According to McKenna (2003) typical barriers to using best evidence include: cost effectiveness where the 'best' practice may be considered more/too expensive; entrenched attitudes where practitioners are reluctant to change current 'practice wisdom'; lack of support from managers or colleagues where the need for best practice is not recognized or prioritized; and lack of time where busy practitioners do not have time to study and reflect on their practice.

User Perspectives as Evidence

Duggan (cited in SPN, 2003b: 1), emphasizes the need for 'shared knowledge and shared territory with a range of disciplines and service users and the general public'. This recognizes users of mental health services and their carers as 'experts by experience' with a right to define their own research agendas. In recent years, more research studies have begun to emerge that are consistent with this approach (see Faulkner and Layzell, 2000; Mental Health Foundation, 2003; Rose, 2001; Samele et al., 2007; Thornicroft et al., 2002). These studies have adopted sound methodological protocols derived from the expanding literature on user- and carer-centred research (Beresford, 2007a). They place a high value on both qualitative methods and dialogistic relationships between researchers and participants. They challenge the presumption of incompetence that has characterized and dominated professional attitudes towards users of mental health services. The mentally distressed and their carers are gradually being recognized as valid contributors to knowledge; their knowledge is being valued and disseminated with the intention of informing the development of policy and practice.

For example, User-Focused Monitoring (UFM) was first developed in 1996 by the Sainsbury Centre for Mental Health. This is a way of carrying out research where people who use mental health services evaluate the experiences of other mental health service users in both community and hospital settings. User-Focused Monitoring puts service users at the heart of the process since they lead each stage of the UFM evaluation process. The first UFM project was carried out in Kensington, Chelsea and Westminster as a pilot project in 1996 (Rose et al., 1998). Since then, many projects have developed around the country that use the term UFM to describe their work. A major piece of research, *Users' Voices: The Perspectives of Mental Health Service Users on Community and Hospital Care* (Rose, 2001), was created, developed, carried out and analysed by a group of mental health service users with severe and enduring mental health problems. Sixty-one trained user interviewers interviewed over 500 service users on seven sites in urban and rural communities and in hospital settings. This study offers a valuable insight into the importance of user-led research in defining standards of good practice in mental health care and categorically demonstrates that people who use services are more than capable of conducting methodologically robust, high quality research.

There is now a substantial and consistent evidence base from service user focused research that challenges the ways in which mental health professionals and researchers have traditionally viewed services and their impact (Davis, cited in SPN, 2004). Professionally driven research has focused on the reduction of symptoms and psychiatric service use as the prime measures of the success of mental health interventions. However, evidence from the service user literature suggests that many users:

> see these as but side issues to their 'real' problems which they locate as being able to participate in society, support themselves and to enjoy feelings of well being. Hence many users of mental health services see their principal needs much as others do – they would value employment, a decent income, decent housing and a chance to make and sustain social relationships. These and symptom reduction are not always mutually exclusive but they may conflict. (Barnes and Bowl, 2001: 95)

It is essential that user-led research is placed on an equal footing with professional research. As Faulkner and Thomas argue, 'a marriage of two types of expertise is the essential ingredient of the best mental health care: expertise by experience and expertise by profession' (2002: 3).

CHAPTER SUMMARY

Professionally-driven bio-medical approaches have dominated the field of mental health treatment, research and evaluation. These have all too often been based on misplaced assumptions about the capacity of the mentally distressed to make meaningful contributions to the knowledge base and this has resulted in them being marginalized from the sites of power in policy and practice. It is evident that the medical model alone is an inadequate basis for effective and acceptable mental health policy and practice. As Duggan states, 'the persistent "medicalisation" of mental health service models and research priorities appears to relate very little to an accompanying evidence base which indicates that advances in pharmacology and other medical treatments have resulted in little consistent improvement in recovery rates' (cited in SPN, 2003b: 1). Clearly a broader evidence base is required. More recently there appears to be a greater willingness to embrace social and experiential perspectives on mental distress alongside traditional psycho-medical approaches, and also to engage with knowledge and evidence emerging from the activities of the mental health service user movement. This is good news and implies a long overdue partnership approach between people who use services, practitioners and researchers towards constructing a solid evidence base for mental health policy and practice.

Further reading/resources

Fennell, P. (1996) *Treatment without Consent: Law, Psychiatry and the Treatment of Mentally Disordered People Since 1845*. London: Routledge.

Moncrieff, J. (2007) *The Myth of the Chemical Cure: a Critique of Psychiatric Drug Treatment*. Basingstoke: Palgrave Macmillan.

Social Perspectives Network (2007) *Whose Recovery is it Anyway?* London: Social Perspectives Network (available at www.spn.org.uk).

6 CHALLENGING INEQUALITY AND RESPECTING DIVERSITY

This chapter can be used to support the development of knowledge and skills in professional social work as follows:

National Occupational Standards for Social Work

Key Role 1: Prepare for and work with individuals, families, carers, groups and communities to assess their needs and circumstances

- Prepare for social work contact and involvement.

Key Role 2: Plan, carry out, review and evaluate social work practice, with individuals, families, carers, groups and communities and other professionals

- Interact with individuals, families, carers, groups and communities to achieve change and development and to improve life opportunities
- Work with groups to promote individual growth, development and independence
- Address behaviour which presents a risk to individuals, families, carers, groups, communities.

Key Role 3: Support individuals to represent their needs, views and circumstances

- Advocate with and on behalf of, individuals, families, carers, groups and communities.

Key Role 6: Demonstrate professional competence in social work practice

- Contribute to the promotion of best social work practice.

(TOPSS England, 2002)

Academic Standards for Social Work

Honours graduates in social work:

4.6 must learn to:

- recognise and work with the powerful links between intrapersonal and interpersonal factors and the wider social, legal, economic, political and cultural context of people's lives

Challenging Inequality and Respecting Diversity

- understand the impact of injustice, social inequalities and oppressive social relations
- challenge constructively individual, institutional and structural discrimination.

4.7 should learn to become accountable, reflective, critical and evaluative which involves learning to:

- think critically about the complex social, political and cultural contexts in which social work is located.

5.1 should acquire, critically evaluate, apply and integrate knowledge and understanding in relation to:

5.1.1 Social work services, service users and carers

- the social processes (associated with, for example, poverty, migration, unemployment, poor health, disablement, lack of education and other sources of disadvantage) that lead to marginalisation, isolation and exclusion and their impact on the demand for social work services
- explanations of the links between definitional processes contributing to social differences (for example, social class, gender, ethnic differences, age, sexuality and religious belief) to the problems of inequality and differential need faced by service users
- the nature and validity of different definitions of, and explanations for, the characteristics and circumstances of service users and the services required by them, drawing on knowledge from research, practice experience, and from service users and carers.

5.5.3 should be able to analyse and synthesise information gathered for problem solving purposes to:

- critically analyse and take account of the impact of inequality and discrimination in work with people in particular contexts and problem situations.

5.6 should be able to communicate clearly, accurately and precisely (in an appropriate medium) with individuals and groups in a range of formal and informal situations, i.e. to:

- listen actively to others, engage appropriately with the life experiences of service users, understand accurately their viewpoint and overcome personal prejudices to respond appropriately to a range of complex personal and interpersonal situations
- communicate effectively across potential barriers resulting from differences (for example, in culture, language and age).

5.7 should be able to work effectively with others, i.e. to:

- involve users of social work services in ways that increase their resources, capacity and power to influence factors affecting their lives
- act with others to increase social justice by identifying and responding to prejudice, institutional discrimination and structural inequality
- challenge others when necessary, in ways that are most likely to produce positive outcomes.

(QAA, 2008)

> **Key themes in this chapter**
>
> - Theorizing inequality and discrimination – Thompson's PCS analysis
> - Understanding inequality and oppression in the lives of the mentally distressed – key diversity issues for mental health practitioners: class; race and ethnicity; gender; sexual orientation; disability; and age.
> - Fighting back – human rights and the mental health user movement
> - Human rights based practice in mental health.

INTRODUCTION

In Chapters 1 and 2 we established that alienating and exclusionary attitudes and practices towards the mentally distressed have a long history and remain firmly embedded in contemporary society. According to the Disability Rights Commission (2007) discrimination and inequality systematically destroy people's mental health. In this chapter we explore further how the dynamics of discrimination and inequality shape the lives of people in mental distress and their experiences of mental health services. We begin by returning to Thompson's personal, cultural and structural (PCS) analysis of the processes that produce and sustain inequalities, discrimination and oppression in society. Key diversity issues for mental health practitioners are highlighted, including: class; race and ethnicity; gender; sexual orientation; disability; and age. We then go on to explore the history of resistance and rights based collective action amongst the mentally distressed and the significance and impact of the mental health service user movement on contemporary mental health policy and practice. Finally, we conclude with a discussion of the need for a human rights based approach in mental health.

THEORIZING INEQUALITY AND DISCRIMINATION

As outlined in Chapter 1, Thompson's (2006) PCS analysis (Figure 6.1) can assist social work practitioners in developing an understanding of how discrimination and inequalities feature in the lives of users of services and in their dealings with welfare systems. Thompson explains how discrimination and inequalities operate at three levels – the personal or psychological (P); the cultural (C) and the structural (S).

The 'P' level represents *personal* thoughts, feelings, attitudes and actions and how these can lead to prejudicial judgements. However, personal discrimination operates within the 'C' level or *cultural* context. Here, shared ways of seeing, thinking and doing (norms and values) are transmitted and reinforced through various societal institutions (including families, religious organizations and the media) producing

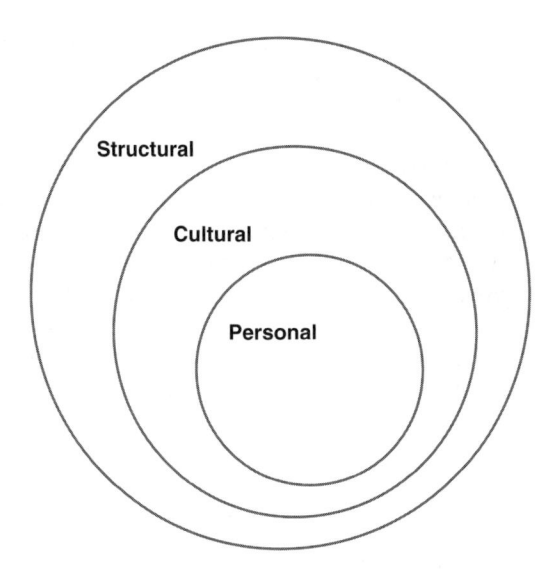

Figure 6.1 Thompson's (2006) PCS Analysis

powerful notions about what is considered 'normal' or 'right'. This enables us to see how classism, racism, sexism, heterosexism, disablism and ageism are more than personal prejudice. They are the manifestations of oppressive and discriminatory culture *through* individual thought or action. Thompson usefully cites Berger to illustrate further:

> Society not only controls our movements, but shapes our identity, our thoughts and emotions. The structures of society become the structure of our own consciousness. Society does not stop at the surface of our skins. Society penetrates us as much as it envelops us. (Berger, cited in Thompson, 2006: 28)

The cultural level is, in turn, embedded within the 'S' level – the *structural*. This is the level of institutionalized, interlocking social divisions and power relations in society – class, race, gender, sexuality, disability and age.

Thompson's PCS analysis enables us to appreciate the complexity of the ways in which discrimination operates in society and how the three levels interact with and reinforce each other. It also enables the individual social worker to develop a sharper awareness of the need for discrimination to be tackled at all three levels, whilst recognizing the limits to her/his capacity to influence change the further s/he is located from the personal level. However, readers of this book would do well to take note of Thompson's warning in his recent reflections on the use of his PCS analysis:

> I have come across many examples of students simply referring to PCS analysis without showing any real understanding of it or how it can be used. It is as if it has become a 'mantra' to be uttered, rather than an analytical framework that can help us make sense

of the complexities of discrimination and oppression. I am concerned to ensure that it should not be used in an unthinking or uncritical way. It should be used as a basis of critically reflective practice not as an alternative to it. (2006: 32)

Thompson's PCS analysis is extremely valuable in providing us with an overarching framework within which we can theorize 'multiple oppressions'. For example, research by Barn (2008) emphasizes the importance of social workers' understanding of the *interconnections* between ethnicity, gender, social class and mental health in order to promote improved policy, provision and practice. Nevertheless, it remains important that practitioners have knowledge and understanding of some of the *specific* ways in which inequalities and discrimination shape the experiences of users of mental health services and we consider some these in the next section.

INEQUALITY AND OPPRESSION IN THE LIVES OF THE MENTALLY DISTRESSED – KEY DIVERSITY ISSUES FOR MENTAL HEALTH PRACTITIONERS

Group reflection exercise

Understanding the law on equality and discrimination

Listed below is a chronology of key anti-discrimination policy and legislation in the UK.

1970 *The Equal Pay Act*
1975 *The Sex Discrimination Act*
1976 *The Race Relations Act*
1995 *The Disability Discrimination Act*
1998 *The Human Rights Act*
2000 *The Race Relations (Amendment) Act*
2001 *The Race Equality Duty*
2004 *The Civil Partnership Act*
2006 *The Equality Act*
      The Disability Equality Duty
2007 *The Equality Act (Sexual Orientation) Regulations*
      The Gender Equality Duty

In small groups discuss the following question:

How can mental health social workers use anti-discrimination policy and legislation effectively in their work?

Despite progressive developments in anti-discrimination and human rights policy and legislation in the UK over the last four decades, research evidence demonstrates that inequalities and discrimination continue to shape the lives of the mentally distressed and are reflected in mental health services in their various forms – class, race, gender, sexual orientation, disability and age. We now explore each of these in turn.

Class

Mental health services are dominated by people from poor backgrounds. Studies have consistently reported the close association between mental distress and poverty (Brown and Harris, 1978; Hollingshead and Redlich, 1958; Meltzer, 1995; Sheppard, 2002; WHO, 1995) though determining which comes first – if being poor renders a person more susceptible to mental distress, or if mental distress pulls a person into poverty – is more difficult to answer. The relationship has long been assumed to be interactive. Research shows that children in families of Social Class V are more likely to have a mental disorder than those in Social Class I (Meltzer et al., 2000). The highest rates of mental disorders among children occur among those from families where no parent has ever worked.

An analysis of the 1999 *Poverty and Social Exclusion Survey* data revealed that 'whilst overall a quarter of PSE respondents were defined as poor, over half of the survey's respondents with mental ill-health were in this group. Poor mental health is disproportionately found amongst the poorest in society' (Payne, 2000: 9). Additionally, Payne notes the increased risk of poor mental health amongst those reporting social exclusion, not only from the labour market, but also from participation in social relationships and other activities that characterize modern life.

While access to paid work usually acts as a protective factor for positive mental health, when it is poorly paid, of low status or carried out in stressful or hazardous conditions, it is a risk factor for negative mental health (WHO, 2004). The mentally distressed are seriously disadvantaged in the labour market and consequently exposed to poverty, ill-health, homelessness and even imprisonment (Sayce, 2000). People with mental health problems are the largest single group of incapacity benefits claimants in the UK. In a survey of the experiences and expectations of almost 2,000 disabled people commissioned by the UK Government's Office for Disability Issues, researchers found that while 43 per cent of respondents of working age were in work, this applied to just 16 per cent of those with a mental health diagnosis (Williams et al., 2008). In its 2008 Green Paper *No One Written Off: Reforming Welfare to Reward Responsibility* the Government announced that it wants to help the one million or more people on incapacity benefits with depression, anxiety and other mental health problems into work. Many mentally distressed people want to work and with the right support and encouragement can do so, however the biggest barriers to work are the stigmatizing attitudes and discriminatory behaviours towards them (Citizen's Advice Bureau, 2004).

In 2008 the Social Policy Research Unit (Sainsbury et al., 2008) investigated the relationship between mental health and employment for the UK Department for Work and Pensions. The researchers found that people were generally reluctant to tell their employer about a mental health condition because of fears of a negative reaction. This and other research findings suggest that these fears are well founded. In the study for the UK Government Office for Disability Issues cited above, 12 per cent of respondents felt they had been treated unfairly or discriminated against because of their impairment. However, this applied to 35 per cent of people with a mental health diagnosis. More than a quarter of people with mental health problems who were of working age felt they had not got a job they had applied for because of their diagnosis, compared to 15 per cent on average (Williams et al., 2008). Research conducted by the UK Government Social Exclusion Unit reported that, despite the provisions of The Disability Discrimination Act 1995, one-third of mentally distressed people had been dismissed or forced to resign from their job (Office of the Deputy Prime Minister, 2004). Almost four in 10 believed that they had been denied a job because of their mental health history, and over two-thirds had been put off applying for jobs for fear of unfair treatment. The research revealed that fewer than one in four employers would consider employing someone with a history of mental health problems. One attempt to address this has been the adoption of a broader definition of 'disability' with the amendment of The Disability Discrimination Act in 2005, so that its provisions now extend to many more mentally distressed people. In addition, all public bodies are now covered by The Disability Equality Duty 2006 which requires public service providers to demonstrate that their practices do not discriminate against disabled people, either as employees or as users of services.

Other discriminatory practices restrict the social opportunities and reduce the financial security of mentally distressed people. For example, people with a mental health diagnosis often have difficulty in obtaining health, travel and life insurance cover from companies even though this is illegal under the Disability Discrimination Act 1995 (Citizen's Advice Bureau, 2004).

Race and Ethnicity

As we established in Chapter 1, what actually constitutes mental health and mental 'disorder' or 'illness' has been the subject of intense debate within Western culture for some time. However, these debates are intensified considerably when we introduce questions of cultural diversity. According to Suman Fernando there is a need to:

> (a) recognize that cultures develop their own norms for health, for ideal states of mind and for what is considered correct functioning of individuals in society; and (b) take on board the fact that the study of these 'cultural' norms may be distorted by prejudiced – often racist – perceptions of the cultures and the people associated with those cultures. (2008: 45)

An examination of the history of psychiatry illustrates how it was saturated with the values, ideologies and assumptions of Western European culture right from the beginning. While racism has existed for centuries, racist stereotypes of non-Western peoples worked their way into the very fabric of mental health theory and practice. Fernando explains how many of these stereotypes originate in the era of colonialism and slavery. For example, some highly influential early psychologists and psychiatrists (for example Freud, 1913; Maudsley, 1867; Pritchard, 1835; Tuke, 1858) subscribed to the idea that non-Europeans were 'savages' with primitive instincts and therefore no capacity for mental distress. Others claimed that black people had an instinct for submission (McDougall, 1920) and would become prey to mental illness if set free from slavery (Cartwright, 1851) (all cited in Fernando, 1995). These pejorative stereotypes have their modern equivalents, for example in the labelling of African Caribbean mental health service users as 'big, black and dangerous'. Clearly, therefore, ethnocentric and racist thinking have always been part of the mental health system (Fernando, 2002).

The inquiry into the death of David Bennett in psychiatric services in 1998 (Norfolk, Suffolk and Cambridgeshire Strategic Health Authority, 2003) concluded that NHS psychiatric services in the UK were institutionally racist.

Key terms (1)

Institutional racism is defined in the report of the inquiry into the police investigation of the murder of the black teenager Stephen Lawrence (the Macpherson Report) as:

'The collective failure of an organisation to provide an appropriate and professional service to people because of their colour, culture or ethnic origin … . It can be seen or detected in processes, attitudes and behaviour that amount to discrimination through unwitting prejudice, ignorance, thoughtlessness and racist stereotyping that disadvantages minority ethnic people'. (Macpherson, 1999: 28)

The key theme underpinning most of the 22 recommendations from the Bennett Inquiry was that there should be ministerial acknowledgement of the presence of institutional racism in the mental health system and a commitment to eliminate it.

Racism within mental health services deters people from trying to access help as soon as they begin to experience distress. In a 2003 survey conducted for the Department of Health, 61 per cent of respondents found that staff racism was a problem within services; while 78 per cent of Black, 61 per cent of Asian, 49 per cent of Irish and 44 per cent of Chinese respondents said that racism among staff was a major hindrance in accessing services (Walls and Sashidharan, 2003). Other research studies have continued to highlight significant shortcomings in the quality of mental health care received by Black and minority ethnic (BME) communities (Commission for Healthcare Audit and Inspection, 2005; NIMHE, 2003; SCMH, 2002). Often a lack of understanding of cultural diversity in the experience and expression of distress leads to the reinforcement of cultural stereotypes which can result in misdiagnosis and negligent care. Black people (particularly African-Caribbean people) are over represented at the 'sharp end' of the mental health system. For example, African Caribbean men, often stereotyped as violent and dangerous, are more likely to be diagnosed with schizophrenia; more likely to be compulsorily detained in psychiatric hospital and more likely to be given high doses of psychoactive medication. They are also more likely to be brought into psychiatric services by the police (Commission for Healthcare Audit and Inspection, 2005; Harrison, 2002; NIMHE, 2003; SCMH, 2002). Research has also shown that individuals from Asian and African-Caribbean origins are more likely to be misunderstood and misdiagnosed and more likely to be prescribed drugs and ECT rather than talking treatments such as psychotherapy and counselling (MIND, 2003b, 2006; Nazroo and King, 2002).

In 2005, in response to increased awareness of racial discrimination in the psychiatric system, the UK Department of Health introduced its Black and Minority Ethnic Mental Health Programme via the National Institute for Mental Health in England.

> **The NIMHE Black and Minority Ethnic Mental Health Programme**
>
> The NIMHE Black and Minority Ethnic Mental Health programme aims to improve the mental health care of all people of Black and minority ethnic (BME) status, including those of Irish or Mediterranean origin and east European migrants. It aims to:
>
> - enhance the quality of life, challenge exclusion through improved mental health services and health outcomes
> - develop appropriate training and support to staff to deliver culturally competent services, with confidence
> - enhance, or build capacity within, BME communities and the voluntary sector to deal with mental health and mental ill health
> - to ensure compliance with statutory obligations: Race Relations (Amendment) Act 2000, Human Rights Act 1998.
>
> (DH, 2005c)

The focus of the Black and Minority Ethnic Mental Health Programme is, as indicated in the title, *Delivering Race Equality in Mental Health Care* – a five-year action plan aimed at reducing inequalities in access to, experience of, and outcomes from mental health services for BME users (DH, 2005c). However while this publication accepted most of the recommendations from the Bennett Inquiry, it rejected the existence of institutional racism in mental health services, preferring to talk of 'direct' and 'indirect' discrimination. In doing so, it ignores the findings of the Macpherson Report and the substantial research evidence available in this area since the 1970s. Furthermore, using Thompson's PCS analysis, we can see that such an approach fails to contextualize the various forms of direct and institutional racism in the wider society. Experiences of racism and disadvantage in all areas of life have a major impact on the mental health of people from black and ethnic minority (BME) backgrounds from unemployment (MIND, 2003b, 2006; ONS, 2004) through to harassment and violence (Fernando, 2003).

Gender

> **Key terms (2)**
>
> **Sexism**: 'A social relationship in which males have authority over females'.
>
> **Patriarchy**: 'A system of male authority which oppresses women through its social, political and economic institutions'.
>
> (Humm, 1995: 200, 258)

The longstanding existence of institutionalized sexism within psychiatry has obscured the need to question the social structures of patriarchy (Coppock, 2008). Consequently, the particular social consequences and experiences of being a woman and its effects on mental health are only recently beginning to be acknowledged in women's mental health care. In a world where women are routinely disadvantaged by gender inequalities this means that they are at much greater risk of being adversely affected by poverty than their male counterparts (Wetzel, 2000). Women in general are poorer and experience greater deprivation; have less social and political power and have less access to health, education and employment than men (WHO, 2001c). Lone mothers and older women are particularly vulnerable to poverty and therefore are at greater risk of mental distress (Bebbington et al., 2002; Doyal, 2000). Research also suggests that older women who have primarily worked within the domestic sphere are more likely to experience depression than those employed outside the home (Milne and Williams, 2003).

Studies in the UK and US reveal that at least half of women using mental health services have experienced sexual or physical abuse as children and/or adults (Itzin, 2006; McCauley et al., 1997; Mullen et al., 1993). Women who have experienced violence, whether in childhood or adult life have increased rates of depression and anxiety, post-traumatic stress disorder, phobias, chemical dependency, substance misuse and suicidal thoughts and behaviour (WHO, 2000, 2001c). Overall there is evidence to suggest that women's mental health could be significantly improved by: gaining control over the determinants of their mental health (in particular eliminating situations where they are devalued and discriminated against); reducing the exposure of women to those risk factors which compromise their mental health (especially violence and abuse); and involving women in decision-making in all aspects of their lives.

Since the 1970s, numerous research studies have explored the ways in which women are treated within psychiatry and psychiatric services (Chesler, 1972; Penfold and Walker, 1984; Showalter, 1987; Ussher, 1991). Women's experiences of mental health care have been found to be overwhelmingly negative with evidence of gender bias and stereotyping in diagnosis and treatment. Mental health professionals have been found to locate problems within women and fail to recognize the socio-political factors outlined above that are often both the context and source of their distress (Broverman et al., 1970; Chesler, 1972; Loring and Powell, 1988; Sheppard, 1991; WHO, 2001c). This has frequently led to women's mental distress being trivialized and their unhappiness explained away as some internal flaw. In a Mind survey (Read and Baker, 1996) 58 per cent of women respondents said that they had been treated unfairly compared to 41 per cent of men. Furthermore, 40 per cent of women and 26 per cent of men complained of unfair treatment from their GPs or of GPs who appeared to lack knowledge of, or interest in, mental distress. Women report that medication is often the only option made available to them (Resisters, 2002; Scott and Williams, 2001) and they are 48 per cent more likely to be prescribed psychotropic medication (Simoni-Wastila, 2000). Older women are over-represented in official statistics recording administrations of ECT (DH, 2002b). The majority of mental health care for women in the UK is located in generic, mixed-sex services. Those women-only services that are available are patchy and usually provided by the voluntary sector. Regarding mental health care in hospital or residential settings, a recurring theme is the risk of abuse or harassment (DH, 2002a). The National Patient Safety Agency identified 19 reported rapes in two years, as well as other sexual assaults (Scobie et al., 2006).

In 2002 the UK Department of Health consulted women service users regarding their experiences of mental health care and some powerful messages emerged both for government and for mental health practitioners. Women reported that:

- They are not listened to, nor are their views taken seriously.
- They want access to services that are designed to empower them, promoting choice and self-determination.
- They need mental health practitioners capable of understanding the underlying causes and context of their mental distress.
- They want recognition of their strengths and abilities as survivors.
- They need to feel safe when receiving mental health care.

Subsequently the government launched its Women's Mental Health Strategy (DH, 2002b, 2003c) to achieve a mainstream approach to gender in mental health service organization and delivery and to ensure that women feel better served by the mental health care systems in terms of their individual experience. The strategy provides a framework for addressing gender inequalities in mental health system. Additionally, from 1 April 2007, there is a legal requirement to demonstrate equity of outcome for women and men in all aspects of policy, workforce issues and service delivery under the Gender Equality Duty introduced as part of the Equality Bill in March 2005 (DTI, 2005). However, for these developments to be truly effective, nothing short of a cultural sea change is required. Evidence drawn from the Department of Health consultation (DH, 2002b) and elsewhere (SPN, 2005) points to a widespread reluctance amongst practitioners to treat gender and other inequalities seriously. This would suggest that the hearts and minds of mental health professionals are still not attuned to the impact of gender inequality on women's mental health, or indeed on their own attitudes and behaviour.

Although women are more likely than men to be treated for a mental health problem, it is also important to recognize that men too are adversely affected by gender stereotyping and inequality in the mental health system. Patriarchal constructions of masculinity as well as femininity may contribute to experiences of mental distress for men. Many men may find it difficult to recognize and seek help for mental distress since this is 'incompatible' with masculinity (Frosh, 1997). Younger men may have become particularly vulnerable in the context of increasing unemployment, occupational uncertainty, widespread substance misuse and family/relationship breakdown (Hawton, 1998, 2000). Recent research paints a picture of young men who are disengaged from both society and mainstream services (Spurrell et al., 2003). With the notable exceptions of China and parts of India, the rate of death by suicide is higher for men than women in almost all parts of the world (although suicide *attempts* remain more common among women than men) (WHO, 2002). Policy initiatives such as the National Suicide Prevention Strategy (DH, 2002c) and Choose Life (Scottish Executive, 2002) have been introduced to specifically target young men. Policy makers and mental health practitioners clearly need to have an awareness of the specific ways in which men talk about and make sense of their emotional distress to ensure an accurate understanding of that distress. Just as with women's mental health, there is a need to move beyond the taken-for-granted constructions of mental health that have detracted from the quality of mental health care to both sexes.

Sexual Orientation

Many of our social and economic institutions have a history of promoting heterosexuality as the norm – the legal system, the armed forces, public services, including health and education, and many religions have histories of institutionalized homophobia (MIND, 2008b). Culturally too, homophobic beliefs and values have been transmitted through traditions and rituals, literature and the arts, and through the mass media. It should come as no surprise then to learn that in the same way that racism and sexism have permeated the knowledge base of the mental health professions, so too have heterosexism and homophobia.

Key terms (3)

Heterosexism: 'bias shown by a society or community where cultural institutions and individuals are conditioned to expect everyone to live and behave as heterosexuals'.

Homophobia: 'the irrational hatred, intolerance and fear of LGB people'.

(Stonewall, www.stonewall.org.uk)

Homophobia was given legitimacy within psychiatry and psychology by theories of mental illness that pathologized homosexuality. The *Diagnostic and Statistical Manual of Mental Disorders* (DSM) of the American Psychiatric Association included homosexuality as a classified mental disorder from 1952 until 1973. Similarly, the World Health Organization's *International Statistical Classification of Diseases and Related Problems* (ICD) only removed homosexuality from its classification system in 1992. Lesbian, gay and bisexual (LGB) people were subjected to damaging attempts to 'cure' them of their sexuality, including hospitalization and aversion therapy (MIND, 2008b).

Obviously, just like heterosexual people, LGB people can experience mental distress but being lesbian, gay or bisexual is not in itself a mental health problem. However, a variety of social factors can affect the lives of LGB people that mean they are likely to experience mental distress (McFarlane, 1998). A wide range of research evidence suggests that LGB people have higher levels of psychological distress than heterosexual people and they are more likely than heterosexuals to have consulted a mental health professional. In particular, anxiety, depression, self-harm and suicidal feelings are more common among LGB people than among heterosexual people, as are high rates of drug and alcohol misuse (King and McKeown, 2003; King et al., 2007; Warner, 2004).

Homophobia can cause the most obvious harm to LGB people through bullying and violent attacks while, perhaps more insidiously, heterosexism can seriously damage self-image and self-esteem (Carr, 2003; Stonewall, 2007). Although the British Social Attitudes Survey demonstrates increasing popular acceptance of same-sex partnerships (at least among younger people), the marginalization of and stigma associated with sexual minorities remains (Park, 2005). For example, LGB young people experience more bullying and victimization than their heterosexual counterparts and the mental health consequences of this are seen in the disproportionately high rate of suicidal thoughts and suicide attempts among this group (Pilkington and D'Augelli, 1995; Rivers, 2000, 2001).

While some of the extreme manifestations of the oppression of sexual minorities in the mental health system may now be rare, and LGB people are legally protected from discrimination from providers of goods and services under The Equality Act (Sexual Orientation) Regulations 2007, evidence suggests that widespread discrimination and negative attitudes towards LGB people still exist within services (Hunt and Fish, 2008; McFarlane, 1998). Research by Warner et al. (2004) highlighted the following key issues for LGB people in mental health services:

- mixed or negative reactions when open about their sexuality with health professionals
- a lack of empathy around sexuality issues on the part of health professionals
- visible discomfort on the part of health professionals, and deliberate attempts to avoid discussing sexuality
- the assumption that all service users are heterosexual
- the assumption that being gay, lesbian or bisexual must be a problem for LGB service users
- a minority of health professionals still make a causal link between homosexuality and mental ill health
- a minority of health professionals still display overt homophobia.

Clearly there is still some way to go in achieving the necessary cultural change that would bring about full equality for LGB people in mental health services (MIND, 2008b).

Disability

> ### Key terms (4)
>
> **Impairment**: 'lacking part or all of a limb, or having a defective limb, organism or mechanism of the body'. (Oliver, 1990: 11)
>
> **Disability**: 'the disadvantage and restriction of activity caused by a contemporary social organisation which takes no or little account of people who have physical impairments and thus excludes them from the mainstream of social activities'. (Oliver, 1990: 11)
>
> **Disablism**: 'discriminatory, oppressive or abusive behaviour arising from the belief that disabled people are inferior to others'. (Scope, www.timetogetequal.org.uk)

Disability and disablism impact on the lives of *all* those in mental distress. The mentally distressed, like other disabled people, share discrimination on the basis of some presumed 'imperfection' of body, mind or emotion:

> The social model of disability – which says that people are disabled not, or not only, by their so-called 'impairment' (that is, physical, mental or emotional difference from the norm), but instead by the barriers and prejudices that society places in their way – becomes a banner under which user/survivors and other disabled people can rally. (Sayce, 2000: 129).

As we have established in Chapters 1 and 5, the medical model intrinsically focuses on people's *deficits* rather than their *strengths* and this reproduces paternalistic, *disabling* responses in health and social care policy and practice. The medical model also tends to focus on discrete clinical conditions and so disabled people often report how mainstream services are geared towards the treatment of their 'disability' rather than themselves as whole persons. This can have particularly serious implications for those who experience multiple impairments:

> When people were asked what they wanted from mental health and physical disability services, they said they wanted to be seen as 'a whole person', with attention paid to both mental health needs and those relating to physical impairment. They wanted services and professionals to communicate and work together, and easy access to flexible services which could address individual needs. Above all, they wanted to be listened to and treated with respect. (Morris, 2004a: 1)

Research findings from the Department for Work and Pensions (2002) demonstrate how physical impairments, learning impairments and mental distress interact. They found that three-quarters of those meeting the Disability Discrimination Act definition of disability had more than one type of impairment, often a physical impairment and a mental health problem. Morris (2004b) illustrates how people with physical impairments are poorly served by mental health services and vice versa, meaning that people experiencing both often 'fall through the cracks' of provision or experience a fragmenting of their needs across services.

Age

Notwithstanding the material realities of both 'immaturity' (in the case of children) and 'old age' (in the case of adults), as Pilgrim, Rogers and Tummey comment, 'we are conceived, we are born, we develop and then we die after a variable period of time [however] the events within and between these stages and even the length of time involved are shaped and influenced by *social* factors' (2008: 108, our emphasis). In the field of mental health essentialist theories of human development and the life course have been saturated with ageist assumptions regarding the mental life and capacities of children and older adults.

Key terms (5)

Ageism: 'Ageism is a set of beliefs originating in the biological variation between people and relating to the ageing process. It is in the actions of corporate bodies, what is said and done by their representatives, and the resulting views that are held by ordinary ageing people, that ageism is made manifest'.

(Bytheway and Johnson, cited in Bytheway, 1995: 14)

In relation to children, traditional theories from developmental psychology and child and adolescent psychiatry have constructed the 'normal' child (Burman, 1994; Donzelot, 1980; Foucault, 1979; Rose, 1979) and by extension the 'abnormal', 'disturbed' or 'disordered' child (Coppock, 1997, 2005). However, critical research has revealed how the process by which children and young people come to the attention of mental health services 'has as much to do with the feelings and behaviour of other people, and with social customs and routines, as with anything happening inside their heads' (Steinberg, cited in Malek, 1991: 44). It must be acknowledged that culture influences the way in which we define a 'normal' or 'deviant' childhood (Timimi, 2005). This is not to suggest that children and young people do not experience mental distress, but rather to challenge both the reliability and appropriateness of the medical model of mental health in shaping our understanding of and responses to their distress. In Western societies all too often children and young people's resistance to adult authority is pathologized, medicalized and 'treated'. Indeed, we have witnessed an accelerated medicalization of children and young people's emotions and behaviour throughout the late twentieth and early twenty-first centuries. Ever-expanding definitional boundaries of 'disorder' have enveloped more and more children and young people, as for example in the massive explosion in the diagnosis and medical treatment of 'conduct disorders' generally and attention deficit hyperactivity disorder in particular (Coppock, 2002; Timimi, 2005).

According to Timimi (2005) the notion of professionals acting 'in the best interests of the child' has been the most abused phrase in modern child welfare discourse in so far as it is frequently used to justify oppressive decision-making in children and young people's lives. Paternalistic and protectionist approaches, however well-meaning, can lead to children and young people being inappropriately propelled into the mental health system with profound implications for their rights and civil liberties. For example, hospitalization on adult wards, segregation outside mainstream institutions and schools away from family and friends, the use of 'restraint', locked rooms and degrading behaviour modification techniques, and treatment with powerful psychoactive medication (Coppock, 1997, 2002, 2005; Malek, 1991). By contrast, a child and young person-centred approach begins with a recognition of, and genuine commitment to creating, conditions that will promote positive mental health. This means understanding the effect of social, political and economic forces on children and young people's lives and combating those factors that contribute to their mental distress such as poverty, homelessness, violence and racism (Mental Health Foundation, 1998, 1999).

Essentialist and ageist assumptions can also inhibit our understanding of older people's mental health. Poor mental health is often seen as an inevitable part of the ageing process. Such a narrow understanding neglects other very important contextual factors that can either militate against or accelerate the development of mental distress. For example, because of cultural stereotypes of 'senility', many people assume that dementia is the most significant mental health problem in old age. However, depression is far more prevalent in older people, affecting 10–15 per cent of those over 65, whereas dementia affects five per cent of those over 65 (MIND, 2005). Moreover, research has demonstrated that the increased incidence of depression among older adults is linked to *social status*, not simply the physical ageing process. Significant correlates include:

- exit from the labour market (forced or planned retirement)
- poverty (Blaxter, 1990; Murphy, 1982)
- institutionalization in residential care homes
- losses of various kinds – bereavement; confiding relationships; friendships; networks; supports
- elder abuse.

FIGHTING BACK: MENTAL HEALTH, HUMAN RIGHTS AND THE MENTAL HEALTH SERVICE USER MOVEMENT

> **Reflection exercise: listening to users' voices**
>
> Collect some historical and contemporary examples of service user accounts of their experiences of the mental health system.
>
> What similarities can you identify in the stories of users over time? What things do users say disempower them? What could and/or should have happened to avoid this disempowerment?

Personal accounts from mental health service users give a vivid picture of the injustices that have all too often characterized psychiatric intervention in their lives. Porter argues, 'the writings of the mad challenge the discourse of the normal, challenge its right to be the objective mouthpiece of the times' (1987a: 3). In England, protests against psychiatric injustices can be traced back to 1620 when the House of Lords received a petition from the inmates of the Bedlam Asylum complaining of their inhumane treatment. In addition to the personal narratives of those such as Louisa Lowe, Urbane Metcalf, John Mitford, Richard Paternoster and John Perceval, there were a number of campaigning organizations comprised of patients and their allies, such as the Alleged Lunatics' Friend Society which was formed in 1845. The focus at this early stage was primarily directed towards individual cases of injustice rather than the treatment of the insane in general. However, this gradually changed, as Porter describes: 'the history of mad people's writing [became] a crescendo of reaction to, and protest against, the dominating presence of the asylum' (1987b: 273). Identifying this 'long history' of user protest enables us to acknowledge an important sense of continuity with the past – the reality of shared struggles spanning centuries.

It was in the context of the social and political struggles of the turbulent 1960s and 1970s that the seeds of the organized mental health user movement that we recognize today were sown. New social movements sprang up throughout the Western world, campaigning for civil and political rights for oppressed groups including women, black people, disabled people, lesbians and gay men. In the mental health field a powerful fusion of academic, professional and political dissidence gave rise to what subsequently became known as the 'anti-psychiatry' movement. In reality 'anti-psychiatry' was an umbrella term that embraced a wide range of political and ideological positions, but those who identified themselves with the label were united in their condemnation of mainstream psychiatric practice and shared a common concern for the rights of mental patients. In this climate of heightened radical consciousness and political activism, the Mental Patients' Union was formed – an organization that according to Crossley (1999) can justifiably be regarded as the originator of organized service user action in the UK. The Mental Patients' Union was succeeded by a number of smaller groups including the Community Organisation for Psychiatric Emergencies (COPE) and the Campaign Against Psychiatric Oppression (CAPO). By the mid-1980s a variety of localized mental health user forums had been established offering mutual support, however, a number of larger networks were also formed that provided a wider national focus, such as the UK Advocacy Network, Survivors Speak Out, the National Voices Network and the Hearing Voices Network (Wallcraft and Bryant, 2003).

Recent surveys indicate that the mental health service user movement is now made up of in excess of 500 active groups, whereas in 1985 there were only around a dozen (Campbell, 2005; Wallcraft and Bryant, 2003). Campbell states, 'the fact that service users now run their own services, educate most groups of mental health workers, even provide a research team at the Institute of Psychiatry ... is an indication of the different type of landscape we are now inhabiting' (2005: 74). Bamber (2004) and Wallcraft and Bryant (2003) provide excellent accounts of the breadth of activities undertaken. People who use services have made inroads into the mental health system that would have been unimaginable 20 years ago and their knowledge and experiences are directly influencing the direction of policy and practice (SCIE, 2008). For example, recent developments around direct payments and personalized budgets for services (see Chapter 3) owe much to the research and campaigning activities of user-led organizations such as Shaping Our Lives and the National Centre for Independent Living.

However, 'this transformation cannot be attributed to service user action alone' (Campbell, 2005: 74). An equally significant 'driver' for user involvement in mental health services has been the ideological shift in government policy and legislation from the late 1980s onwards that brought unprecedented structural change in health and welfare services. The NHS and Community Care Act 1990 introduced a market-oriented approach and the application of general management principles into the design and delivery of health and welfare services, disrupting the traditional balance of power between clinicians and 'their' patients. The managerialist approach emphasizes the centrality of 'consumer choice' and 'user involvement' in the design, delivery and evaluation of mental health services and this has been a prominent theme in government policy and legislation for the last two decades. The consumerist emphasis on choice and the importance of professionals being accountable to users of their services certainly chimes with the longstanding concerns of mental patients about their treatment in the system. However, it must be remembered that consumerist discourse reflects profoundly different political, economic and ideological priorities to the discourse of user empowerment. The philosophy and activities of the mental health service user movement are rooted in historical and enduring experiences of collective struggle and resistance to social injustice, oppression and discrimination – essentially the language of human rights, not that of consumerism.

This has led some commentators to express concern about the capacity of oppressive systems to hijack the language of rights to convey a powerful illusion of inclusivity, participation and empowerment (see for example Rose, 1986). From this perspective it could be argued that rather than empowering the mentally distressed, there is a danger that government agendas around user involvement may simply reorganize relations between mental health professionals and service users to the extent that radicalism is effectively neutralized. User organizations must be mindful of the scope for their activities to become incorporated into an oppressive system rather than challenging and disrupting the power relations within it. Indeed, for the majority of the mentally distressed, consumerism has done very little to challenge the persistence of professional (and especially medical) hegemony in the mental health system. For the most part, mental health professionals still have the power to decide what services will be made available and to whom. As we established in Chapters 3 and 4, real choice of treatments for mental distress remains illusive; is almost always mediated through care managers and is constrained by the rationing of scarce state resources. The government's 'personalization agenda' has the *potential* to bring about a fundamental shift of power towards service users. Individual budgets and self assessments will, theoretically, enable them to have greater choice and control over the support they receive. However, if personalization is to become more than just another piece of government rhetoric, then it has to be informed by a rights-based approach. As Peter Beresford points out:

> you have to adopt the right core values. It is more than just having a whole manual of different tools to use: it is about thinking in a different way, starting with the person, not the service. For service users, person-centred support is based on trust and honesty, the relationship that we have with practitioners. For practitioners, it means building a relationship in which people feel as though their self-esteem and their self-awareness are raised to think about what they want, because maybe that is something they have never really been asked. (*The Guardian,* 23 July 2008)

HUMAN RIGHTS BASED PRACTICE IN MENTAL HEALTH

> Social work is, by nature, holistic in approach and views the individual within a wider context of their personal, familial, cultural and socio-economic circumstances. Its ethos is on empowerment and promoting independence through a focus on 'working with' rather than 'doing to' which helps to increase personal achievement, self-fulfilment and create a much stronger sense of citizenship. (Joannides, cited in SPN, 2004: 14)

Social work has a longstanding commitment to social justice issues and principles of promoting independence, dignity, choice and self determination amongst users of services and their carers. The centrality of anti-discriminatory and anti-oppressive theory and practice in social work education and training means that social workers are highly attuned to issues of power, oppression and social exclusion. It also means that they develop a critical awareness of their own potential for oppression towards users and carers (SCIE, 2008). If mental health services are to become truly user and carer-centred then it is vital that these core professional social work values are not only maintained but also transported into the interprofessional context. This issue is discussed more fully in Chapter 7.

There are some positive developments emerging that give cause for optimism. The British Institute of Human Rights has been working with the Department of Health and a number of NHS organizations to promote the language and practice of human rights in mental health care (DH, 2008g). The intention is to ensure that the core values of Fairness, Respect, Equality, Dignity and Autonomy, better known as the FREDA principles, are at the heart of service provision. A human rights based approach (HRBA) is a way of ensuring that human rights principles and standards are made real in practice (DH, 2008g: 35).

> ### The 5 key HRBA principles
>
> *Principle 1*: Putting human rights principles and standards at the heart of policy and planning.
> *Principle 2*: Ensuring accountability.
> *Principle 3*: Empowerment.
> *Principle 4*: Participation and involvement.
> *Principle 5*: Non-discrimination and attention to vulnerable groups.
>
> (DH, 2008g)

As with the personalization agenda, this approach has the *potential* to transform relationships between mental health professionals and people who use services and their carers. However, real success will depend on the much wider project of eliminating inequality, discrimination and oppression in the lives of the mentally distressed at *personal*, *cultural* and *structural* levels.

CHAPTER SUMMARY

Mental health service users are typically the most vulnerable and powerless in society. We have seen how mental distress can derive from social injustice and oppression and how people experiencing mental distress also face social exclusion and discrimination as a direct consequence of their difficulties. The mandate for robust anti-discriminatory and anti-oppressive practice in the mental health field has been clearly articulated within policy, legislation and by the service user movement for some considerable time. However, it is clear from the evidence cited in this chapter that it is sadly still the case that inequality, discrimination and oppression remain entrenched in the structure and organization of mental health service delivery. Recent developments around human rights based approaches offer some potential for progress to be made, but meaningful change in the lives of the mentally distressed will only come about when their disadvantaged position is acknowledged and addressed at personal, cultural and structural levels.

Further reading/resources

Rogers, A. and Pilgrim, D. (2003) *Mental Health and Inequality*. Basingstoke: Palgrave Macmillan.

Sayce, L. (2000) *From Psychiatric Patient to Citizen. Overcoming Discrimination and Social Exclusion*. Basingstoke: Macmillan.

Thompson, N. (2006) *Anti-discriminatory Practice,* 4th edn. Basingstoke: Palgrave Macmillan.

www.equalityhumanrights.com – Equality and Human Rights Commission.

www.shapingourlives.org.uk – Shaping Our Lives.

7 CROSSING CULTURES
Interprofessional working in mental health

This chapter can be used to support the development of knowledge and skills in professional social work as follows:

National Occupational Standards for Social Work

Key Role 2: Plan, carry out, review and evaluate social work practice, with individuals, families, carers, groups and communities and other professionals.

Key Role 5: Manage and be accountable, with supervision and support, for your own social work practice within your organisation

- Work within multi-disciplinary and multi-organisational teams, networks and systems.

(TOPSS England, 2002)

Academic Standards for Social Work

Honours graduates in social work:

5.1 should acquire, critically evaluate, apply and integrate knowledge and understanding in relation to:

5.1.1 Social work services, service users and carers

- the relationship between agency policies, legal requirements and professional boundaries in shaping the nature of services provided in interdisciplinary contexts and the issues associated with working across professional boundaries and within different disciplinary groups.

5.1.2 The service delivery context

- the significance of interrelationships with other related services, including housing, health, income maintenance and criminal justice (where not an integral social service).

5.1.3 Values and ethics

- the conceptual links between codes defining ethical practice, the regulation of professional conduct and the management of potential conflicts generated by the codes held by different professional groups.

5.1.5 The nature of social work practice

- the factors and processes that facilitate effective interdisciplinary, interprofessional and interagency collaboration and partnership.

5.7 should be able to work effectively with others, i.e. to:

- act co-operatively with others, liaising and negotiating across differences such as organisational and professional boundaries and differences of identity or language
- develop effective helping relationships and partnerships with other individuals, groups and organisations that facilitate change.

(QAA, 2008)

Code of Practice for Social Care Workers

Social care workers have a responsibility for:

6.5 working openly and co-operatively with colleagues and treating them with respect

6.7 recognising and respecting the roles and expertise of workers from other agencies and working in partnership with them.

(General Social Care Council, 2002)

Key themes in this chapter

- New Labour's policy drive towards integrated services and interprofessional practice
- Modernizing mental health services
- Workforce development: new ways of working, new types of worker
- Interprofessional education and training
- Interprofessional working in mental health: messages from research
- Acknowledging tensions between different mental health professionals
- The distinctive contribution of social work in mental health services
- What do service users and carers want from integrated mental health teams?

INTRODUCTION

Bringing together the different skills, knowledge and experience of professionals and others is now considered to be the most effective way of promoting the recovery of those in mental distress. Indeed, interprofessional working is an expectation within the modern mental health system in the UK, underpinned by a plethora of policy directives, legislation and practice guidance. However, while the mandate for such an approach appears to be clear, as ever, in the real world of practice things are not so straightforward. There is now an established research literature documenting, evaluating and analysing the experiences of interprofessional working in the UK and beyond. The messages from this literature are mixed, with examples of interprofessional approaches to service delivery that have been successful and others where it has proved almost impossible to achieve.

In this chapter we provide an overview of the policy developments that underpin the drive towards interprofessional working in mental health. We identify some of the different approaches to interprofessional working that have emerged over the last decade and consider the implications for workforce development, education and training. We highlight some of the messages emerging from recent research studies on interprofessional working and go on to examine the tensions that often exist between mental health professionals that can undermine effective teamwork. Finally, we discuss the challenges currently facing social workers in integrated mental health teams and consider the distinctive contribution of social workers to high quality user and carer-centred mental health care.

Reflection exercise

Why do you think it is important that mental health social workers work closely with other mental health professionals?

MAKING SENSE OF THE POLICY DRIVE TOWARDS INTERPROFESSIONAL PRACTICE

A Note on Terminology

A wide range of terms are currently used to describe the process of working with other professions. These include: working together; joint working; interagency working; interdisciplinary working; interprofessional working; multidisciplinary working; multiprofessional working; collaborative working; partnership; and integrated working. These terms are often used interchangeably, but, as Whittington (2003) advises, there are important distinctions that can be drawn between and within them according to the context in which they are used. For example, 'multidisciplinary team working' is more often used to refer to two or more professionals, agencies or organizations working together where resources, responsibilities and professional expertise are shared through formal or informal partnership arrangements but where professional and/or organizational identities are usually retained. Integrated working, on the other hand, implies a single organizational system of needs assessment, service commissioning and/or service provision, uniting mission, culture, management, budgets, office accommodation, administration and records (Integrated Care Network, 2008).

In similar vein, 'partnership' can refer to a set of formal arrangements entered into by two or more agencies or organizations to provide a service and/or it can simply refer to a value position or principle for practice whereby a professional is committed to working 'in partnership' with other professionals, users of services and their carers. The Social Care Institute for Excellence acknowledges that 'conceptual hybridity and confusion about partnership are rife in the theoretical literature' and in its review of *The Learning, Teaching and Assessment of Partnership Work in Social Work Education*, 'a single, unambiguous definition of partnership work did not emerge' (SCIE, 2006: xi). Clearly then, it is important that we recognize the scope for ambiguity in the meaning and use of these various terms as we engage with the literature on this subject.

New Labour's 'Modernisation Agenda'

Efforts to encourage greater coordination between health and social care systems have been evident in UK government policy since the 1960s. However the NHS and Community Care Act 1990 was the first major step towards achieving this aim. It was intended that the fragmentation that characterized people's experiences of services would be reduced by: (i) a focus on the individual; (ii) the systematic assessment of need, planning and review; (iii) the clarification of agency roles, responsibilities and objectives and an emphasis on effective collaboration. However, as discussed in Chapter 3, the 1990 Act promised a great deal more than it delivered in terms of coordinated approaches to health and social care and significant limitations remained in practice throughout the 1990s.

Since the election of the New Labour government in 1997 the landscape of public service provision in the UK has altered dramatically both in terms of organizational structures and frontline practice. In the context of its 'Modernisation Agenda', the government announced a major programme of reform aimed at achieving 'joined up' public services. In the health and social care field, the continued fragmentation of services between and within organizations and between different professions was seen by New Labour as a major obstacle to effective care:

> All too often when people have complex needs spanning both health and social care good quality services are sacrificed for sterile arguments about boundaries. When this happens, people, often the most vulnerable in our society and those who care for them, find themselves in the no man's land between health and social services. This is not what people want or need. It places the needs of the organisation above the needs of the people they are there to serve. It is poor organisation, poor practice, poor use of taxpayers' money – it is unacceptable. (DH, 1998b: 3)

New powers, or 'flexibilities' were proposed whereby agencies could work more closely together by pooling parts of their budgets, integrating their service provision and/or nominating a lead agency to commission all health and social care services for particular user groups. These proposals were enacted in the Health Act 1999 which placed a statutory duty of partnership on the NHS and Local Authority Social Services Departments.

> ### The Health Act flexibilities
>
> *Pooled budgets*: allows health and local authorities to 'pool' resources into a joint budget which can be accessed by all partners for the commissioning and provision of services.
>
> *Lead commissioning*: allows one authority to delegate functions and transfer funding to the other who will then take responsibility for commissioning health and social care services.
>
> *Integrated provision*: allows for the creation of a single integrated organization providing health and social care.

The *NHS Plan* (DH, 2000) introduced a new type of organization – the Care Trust – to commission and to provide both health and social care:

> The NHS will develop partnerships and co-operation at all levels of care – between patients, their carers and their families and NHS staff; between the health and social care sector; between different government departments; between the public sector, voluntary organisations and private providers in the provision of NHS services to ensure a patient-centred service. (DH, 2000: 5)

The Transition Towards Integrated Services

While coordinated or partnership approaches to service delivery have been developing apace in line with government policy and are recognized as beneficial to users of services and their carers, ultimately it is the *integration* of services (and the work of professionals) in a single organizational system of needs assessment, service commissioning and/or service provision that New Labour believes is the means by which better outcomes can be delivered to the public. This is because, despite the best efforts of those involved, coordinated or partnership arrangements remain essentially fragile and can be difficult to sustain over time. For example, the child protection system in the UK has had a strong tradition of high level interagency collaboration for many years, yet catastrophic communication failures have still occurred, as witnessed so forcefully in the cases of Victoria Climbié and 'Baby P' in the London Borough of Haringey. Following the inquiry into the death of Victoria Climbié the Government concluded that a single organizational structure could address such inherent weaknesses in the system, and set

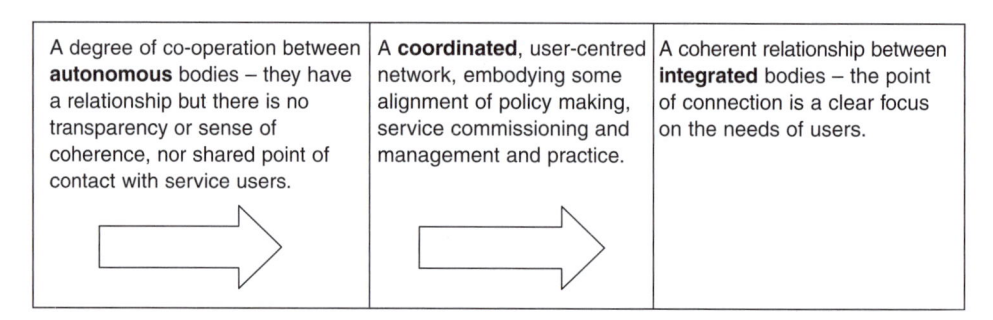

A degree of co-operation between **autonomous** bodies – they have a relationship but there is no transparency or sense of coherence, nor shared point of contact with service users.	A **coordinated**, user-centred network, embodying some alignment of policy making, service commissioning and management and practice.	A coherent relationship between **integrated** bodies – the point of connection is a clear focus on the needs of users.

Figure 7.1

about the wholesale restructuring and integration of services to children, young people and their families through *Every Child Matters* (DH, 2003d), The Children Act 2004 and *The Children's Plan* (DCSF, 2007).

In similar vein, the Green Paper *Independence, Well-being and Choice* signalled the government's plans for transforming adult social care where 'radically different ways of working, redesign of job roles and reconfiguration of services' were to be developed (DH, 2005c: 11–13). These ideas were reinforced in the White Paper *Our Health, Our Care, Our Say* (DH, 2006) which described the government's vision for the development of a holistic, personalized approach to the delivery of social care. The framework for cross-sector reform is set out in the ministerial concordat *Putting People First: a Shared Vision and Commitment to the Transformation of Adult Social Care* (DH, 2007a).

The Integrated Care Network (2008) offers a useful typology mapping the transition in the culture of organizational and professional relationships in UK public services from autonomy, through co-ordination, towards the goal of integration (see Figure 7.1).

Reflection exercise

One of the consistent messages from inquiries into tragedies in both health and social care and child protection is the issue of the various agencies failing to work together.

Why do you think working together is so difficult to achieve in practice? What measures could be introduced to address this?

MODERNIZING MENTAL HEALTH SERVICES

The sheer volume and interconnectedness of government documents relating to the 'joining up' of public services over the last decade makes it difficult to trace a neat chronology of how the changes have developed specifically in relation to mental health policy, legislation and practice. Nevertheless, we can see how, since 1997, the government has set out a number of interlocking pieces of policy which together aim to establish integrated mental health care.

> **Key documents promoting integrated mental health care**
>
> - *Building Bridges: A Guide to Arrangements for Inter-Agency Working for the Care and Protection of Severely Mentally Ill People* (DH, 1995)
> - *Partnership in Action: New Opportunities for Joint Working Between Health and Social Services – A Discussion Document* (DH, 1998b)
> - *Modernising Mental Health Services: Safe, Sound and Supportive* (DH, 1998a)
> - *Effective Care Co-ordination: Modernising the Care Programme Approach* (DH, 1999b)
> - *The National Service Framework for Mental Health: Modern Standards and Service Models* (DH, 1999a)
> - *The NHS Plan: a Plan for Investment, a Plan for Reform* (DH, 2000)
> - *The Mental Health Policy Implementation Guide* (DH, 2001a)
> - *The Ten Essential Shared Capabilities: A Framework for the Whole of the Mental Health Workforce* (DH, 2004)
> - *Independence, Well-being and Choice: Our Vision for the Future of Adult Social Care for Adults in England* (DH, 2005b)
> - *Our Health, Our Care, Our Say: A New Direction for Community Services* (DH, 2006)
> - *Putting People First: A Shared Vision and Commitment to the Transformation of Adult Social Care* (DH, 2007a)
> - *New Ways of Working in Mental Health* (DH, 2007c)
> - *Creating an Interprofessional Workforce: An Education and Training Framework for the Health and Social Care Workforce in England* (DH, 2007d)

As discussed in Chapter 3 the introduction of the Care Programme Approach in 1991 provided a framework for the care of those in mental distress outside hospital, in the community, and required health and local authorities to work together. By the mid-1990s significant overlap had been identified in the operation of the Care Programme Approach and the care management system that had been introduced in local authorities following the NHS and Community Care Act 1990 (DH, 1995). Subsequently, both systems were integrated and updated to avoid confusion for users of services and their carers and to support the new *National Service Framework for Mental Health (NSFMH)* (DH, 1999a; 1999b). For New Labour the implementation of the integrated Care Programme Approach was clearly linked to the development of effective multidisciplinary teams within flexible organizational structures designed to meet the complex needs of those in mental distress.

The *NSFMH* was intended to provide a strategic overview and direction for service improvement in mental health, one of its guiding principles being that 'care will be coordinated between all staff and agencies' (DH, 1999a: 4). Arrangements for enhanced collaboration and coordination between health and social care providers was facilitated through the introduction of the Health Act Flexibilities in 1999 and the *NHS Plan* (DH, 2000), as outlined above. *The Mental Health Policy Implementation Guide* (DH, 2001a) was introduced to support the implementation of the ideas outlined in the *NHS Plan* and the *NSFMH*. It gave detailed descriptions of service models for the different elements of the mental health service including: crisis resolution; assertive outreach; early intervention; primary care and mental health promotion. A 'whole systems' approach was encouraged that would involve 'looking within services to underpinning systems and strategies and ensuring that they support the new pattern of services' and that would require 'new ways of working' (DH, 2001a: 8).

Subsequently, the transition towards integrated Mental Health Care Trusts and Partnership Trusts has been a highly complex affair with some significant variations in arrangements. However, in the main it has been the NHS that has taken the role of lead agency in the provision of mental health services with the most common model of delivery being the co-location of health and social care staff within community teams. Membership of Community Mental Health Teams (CMHTs) typically includes psychiatrists, mental health nurses, social workers, clinical psychologists and occupational therapists (although, as we discuss in the next section, a variety of new roles have been created in recent years). Psychiatrists, nurses, psychologists and occupational therapists are employed by the NHS while social workers are either (i) seconded from their employing local authority to the 'host' NHS trust (that is they are still employed by the local authority but for operational purposes are responsible to the NHS), or (ii) employed directly by the trust. Research has revealed that these arrangements are not without their problems, particularly for social workers who may face significant changes to their terms and conditions of employment and/or may feel isolated from social work colleagues (NIMHE, 2006).

McCrae et al. (cited in Foster, 2005) identified three different models underpinning the management of social work in CMHTs. First a 'traditional' approach, arguing for the rights and empowerment of clients from a sociological stance, with strong links to the local authority and other branches of social work; second an 'eclectic' approach demonstrating an enthusiasm for multidisciplinary teamwork and reducing boundaries between roles, but keen to preserve professional diversity; and finally a 'generic' approach where there is a belief in interdisciplinary working, reducing role demarcation and removing statutory differences where appropriate, and working towards a generic mental health practitioner. The latter 'generic' model has caused particular anxiety for many social workers who are concerned that the essence of the social work contribution to mental health services is at risk of being lost (NIMHE, 2006). These tensions and anxieties will be discussed towards the end of this chapter.

WORKFORCE DEVELOPMENT – NEW WAYS OF WORKING, NEW TYPES OF WORKER

The strong policy drive towards integrated practice has been accompanied by an equally strong drive for workforce reform. Workforce planning has been an expectation in mental health since the publication of the *NSFMH* in 1999, while the *NHS* Plan (DH, 2000) pointed to the need for capacity building in the mental health workforce. A National Workforce Action Team was created within the National Institute for Mental Health in England (NIMHE) to map both the demand for and types of staff that would be needed to support the modernization programme. The New Ways of Working (NWW) programme began in 2003 forming one part of the National Workforce Programme. Initially the focus was on reviewing the role of the consultant psychiatrist (DH, 2005d; National Steering Group, 2004), but it has since been developed to include the whole of the mental health workforce and service users and carers (DH, 2007e). New Ways of Working promotes a 'distributed responsibility' model of working – that is, where responsibility is distributed amongst team members rather than through the consultant psychiatrist as has traditionally been the case. The intention of NWW is to produce a cultural shift in the system whereby those practitioners with the most experience and skills are freed up to work with those with the most complex needs while supervising and supporting other staff to undertake less complex or more routine work. It is argued that this enables existing qualified staff to extend their roles and provides opportunities for new roles to be developed.

A number of new roles have subsequently been developed at the national level, including: Support, Time and Recovery (STR) workers; graduate Primary Care Mental Health Workers; Community Development Workers for BME Communities; and Carer Support Workers. Other new roles designed to help meet specific skills gaps and recruitment needs have been introduced at the local level, such as: Assistant and Associate Mental Health Practitioners; Psychology Associates; Case Managers; and Peer Supporters. Many of these new roles do not require a traditional professional qualification, attracting criticism from some quarters that NWW may be undermining the roles of professionals and/or 'dumbing down' the workforce. Again, we will return to these concerns with particular reference to social work towards the end of this chapter.

The Creating Capable Teams Approach (CCTA) (DH, 2007f) has been developed to support the introduction and implementation of NWW and the new roles and to ensure that multidisciplinary teams focus on the needs of service users and carers. It is a toolkit that engages teams of mental health practitioners and managers from statutory, voluntary and independent sectors and service users and carers in a structured process of reflection on the team's function, the needs of service users and carers, the current workforce structure, and current and required capabilities within the team. The outcomes of these deliberations are recorded and then fed into the workforce planning process.

INTERPROFESSIONAL EDUCATION AND TRAINING

The transition in government policy towards integrated practice and the concomitant changes in workforce development have also had significant implications for professional education and training. Both the integration of health and social care organizations and of social work children's services with education services in local authorities have been important drivers for the development of interprofessional education (IPE). The Laming Report into the circumstances surrounding the death of Victoria Climbié stated:

> The skills involved in working successfully across organisational boundaries must be given proper recognition in both the basic training and in the continuing training of staff. It cannot be left only to those individuals who have the motivation to do it. Working across boundaries should be an expectation placed on all staff, and it must be reflected in training programmes. (Laming, 2003: para 17.113)

Interprofessional education is 'being woven into the fabric of uniprofessional education at the pre-qualifying stage and multiprofessional education at the post-qualifying stage' (Barr and Ross, 2006: 98). As outlined at the beginning of this chapter, both the *National Occupational Standards for Social Work* (TOPSS England, 2002) and the *Subject Benchmark Statement: Social Work* (QAA, 2008) contain explicit statements regarding the importance of teaching, learning and assessment in 'collaborative practice' and 'partnership working' across professional disciplines and agencies. However, as with the tensions surrounding the terminology used to describe working together with other professions outlined above, it is important to recognize the variation and nuances in the terms used to describe the experience of learning with and from other professionals – for example, common learning; shared learning; multiprofessional education and interprofessional education. The definitions given by the UK Centre for the Advancement of Interprofessional Education (CAIPE) (www.caipe.org.uk) are:

- *Multiprofessional education* (may also be referred to as 'shared learning' or 'common learning'): occasions when two or more professions learn side-by-side for whatever reason.
- *Interprofessional education*: occasions when two or more professions learn from and about each other to improve collaboration and the quality of care.

Opportunities for learning with other professionals can range from attending one-off lectures with students from other programmes on a common area of the curriculum, through to studying on a fully integrated interprofessional programme.

Through initiatives such as the *Creating an Interprofessional Workforce Programme* (DH, 2007d), IPE is increasingly being incorporated into mainstream professional education and training for health and social care workers as a means to encourage effective collaborative practice and to improve outcomes for users of services. However, a systematic review of the impact of IPE on professional practice and health care outcomes (Reeves et al., 2008) failed to find sufficiently robust evidence from which to draw any generalizable conclusions about its effectiveness.

The identification and development of core skills and knowledge to support integrated practice is another crucial dimension influencing professional education and training. Integrated frameworks of knowledge, skills and values have been developed as, for example, in the *Capable Practitioner Framework* (SCMH, 2000a) and the *Ten Essential Shared Capabilities* (DH, 2004) for the mental health workforce.

The ten essential shared capabilities for mental health practice

1. Working in partnership
2. Respecting diversity
3. Practising ethically
4. Challenging equality
5. Promoting recovery
6. Identifying people's needs and strengths
7. Providing user centred care
8. Making a difference
9. Promoting safety and positive risk taking
10. Personal development and learning.

(DH, 2004)

The development of the *Ten Essential Shared Capabilities* 'effectively mainstreams a set of values into mental health training with which social workers can immediately identify' (Foster, 2005: 3). Furthermore, social work education and training has long equipped social workers with knowledge, skills and values that are highly valued by users of services:

> The competent social worker [has] a good grasp of sociology, social policy, the law, anti-oppressive and anti-discriminatory practice and individual and group psychology, combined with a mature understanding of how the systems interact. With this underpinning knowledge they are able to bring sound social science and legal knowledge to the team ... . Studies have found that social workers both arrange for services and are a service themselves, providing emotional support and counselling, a range of practical services, and a well-respected advocacy function – carried out with friendliness, openness and professionalism. This is the social worker's technical skill, a less measurable intervention than administering medication but just as valid. (Foster, 2005: 6)

INTERPROFESSIONAL WORKING IN MENTAL HEALTH: MESSAGES FROM RESEARCH

The extrapolation and analysis of key findings from research studies is a necessary and valuable process, informing our understanding of 'what works' and 'what doesn't work' in interprofessional teams. Nevertheless, as discussed in Chapter 5, we have to recognize the enormous complexities involved in researching and evaluating mental health practice, making it difficult (even at times impossible) to make generalizations. As Onyett warns, 'the range of factors at the individual, group, organizational and wider environmental levels that may influence effectiveness are vast and it is difficult to abstract the key elements of team performance that will produce positive outcomes in any given context' (2003: 51).

Research by Borrill et al. (2000) and Norman and Peck (1999) identified certain factors that promote or impede effective interprofessional collaboration in mental health teams. Factors that promoted effective interprofessional working included:

- shared understanding of each other's cultures, roles, responsibilities and methods of working
- direct and regular contact between those providing care
- good communication systems
- individuals with a shared vision and commitment to collaboration underpinned by good management support for innovation
- organizational structures that support interagency collaboration
- national policies that promote and adequately resource coordinated approaches to service delivery.

Factors that impeded effective interprofessional working included:

- lack of a clear and shared vision
- lack of agreement about what working together means
- underdeveloped understanding of each other's roles
- professional protectionism and pursuit of individual professional interests
- ideological differences that inform conflicting models of care
- hierarchical arrangements between health and social care organizations
- separate systems (e.g. information; communication)
- single professional training and preparation for practice
- mistrust of managerial solutions to interprofessional working
- loss of faith in the mental health system.

Additionally, various research studies have reported a range of advantages to be gained from interprofessional working (see, for example, Cook et al., 2001; Gilbert, 2003; Gulliver, 1999; Millar, 2000; Opie, 1997; Peck et al., 2002; Preston et al., 1999; SCMH, 2000b). These include:

- pooled knowledge
- enhanced creativity, skill-mix and skill sharing
- professional development/satisfaction/stimulation
- improved quality of care for users and carers
- single point of contact/easier for users, carers and referrers to negotiate
- efficient use of scarce resources
- more cohesive and congruent management and service delivery
- minimizes bureaucracy and duplication
- easier to 'get things done'.

These upbeat messages are counter-balanced by research studies that reveal significant scepticism regarding the willingness and ability of health and social care professionals to fully engage in the integration process (Allcock, 2003; Hudson, 2002). Research by Stark et al. reported that when budgets are tight and workloads high then 'multiprofessional team working can be scarce in reality' and 'may be Utopian in vision' (2002: 185). Moreover, they concluded that 'there was little evidence ... that multidisciplinary, multiagency approaches actually benefit the user directly and indirectly' (2002: 185). Similarly, the Audit Commission published a very strong critique of partnership working and concluded 'local public bodies should be much more critical about this form of working; it may not be the best solution in every case' (2005: 2). Overall, opinion is mixed about the benefits of current CMHT provision with Webber commenting that, 'they have been surprisingly under-evaluated', with 'case management not faring too well in randomized controlled trials' and that 'systematic reviews of trials of crisis resolution and home treatment (CRHT) teams have not produced definitive results' (2008: 39).

UNCOMFORTABLE BEDFELLOWS? ACKNOWLEDGING THE TENSIONS BETWEEN MENTAL HEALTH PROFESSIONALS

While integrated models of service delivery between health and social care agencies and interprofessional workforce development sound attractive in theory, they may well prove to be heavily problematic in practice. Health and social care professionals have long eyed each other with mutual suspicion. To a certain extent it could be argued that this is due to a lack of understanding of what each profession can bring to the care and treatment of the mentally distressed. However, there are more fundamental differences between the two professional cultures that may militate against harmonious integration. The tensions between the medical and social models of mental health are most forcefully played out in the uncomfortable relationship between social workers and health practitioners. Daisy Bogg (2007) observes unhelpful 'misunderstandings and professional preciousness on both sides', but notes 'social work staff within trusts have a fear and loathing of being in the NHS. The new management structure and the dominance of the medical model are just two of the many areas where anxiety is rife, and the call of "losing professional identity" is common' (2007: 1). Research by Huxley et al. (2005a) reported high levels of stress amongst mental health social workers due to overwork, vacant posts, lack of access to resources, and the pressures associated with constant change and reorganization. Foster (2005) also points to professional isolation and lack of supervision and resources. Huxley et al. (2005b) argue it is essential that the numbers of mental health social workers are maintained in order to ensure that integrated services are genuinely multidisciplinary. Social workers fear that if the new structures continue to be dominated by the traditions and culture of health, with its over-reliance on the medical model – a context that has to date not served users of mental health services well – then their capacity to remain independent may be seriously compromised; especially if they are employed by the same Health Trust as the medical staff. As discussed in Chapter 4, the replacement of the role of Approved Social Worker with that of the Approved Mental Health Professional following the introduction of the Mental Health Act 2007 has caused particular concern:

You're going to have community psychiatric nurses and OTs who are from the same medical model and who will find it hard to take a non-medical view ... [when] the social worker is employed by a different authority and comes from a different professional background, they find it easier to go against a consultant's view than someone who is from within the same organisation. If all three are from the same profession, then multidisciplinary working will not be as effective. (McLean cited in Leason, 2004: 30)

Many mental health social workers fear that the *social* dimension of mental health care is at risk of being lost at precisely the time when it is most urgently needed to inform the development of service user and carer-centred approaches in professional mental health education, training and practice (Tew, 2005). As we discussed in Chapter 5, the current emphasis is on a professional value base that promotes dignity, human worth and social justice and this approach is at the heart of mental health social work.

Reflection exercise

How do you think the historical status differences that get in the way of integrated working in mental health might be overcome?

In November 2005 a Discussion Paper entitled *The Social Work Contribution to Mental Health Services: the Future Direction* was distributed by the NIMHE National Workforce Programme Social Care Group:

to generate a debate with commissioners, employers and social workers in primary, secondary and tertiary MH and social care services on the contribution that social workers can and do make to the support and recovery of people of all ages in mental distress, both now and in the future. (NIMHE, 2006: 2)

A key finding arising from this exercise was that 'social workers promote a unique holistic, recovery orientated, values based social care/social inclusion model that is able to challenge the dominant, task orientated medical model and this is reflected in the competences required. This model should continue in the future' (NIMHE, 2006: 3). Subsequently, as referred to in Chapter 1, the New Ways of Working for Social Work Sub Group identified the distinctive characteristics of social work and the practice capabilities of social workers in interdisciplinary teams (see below). By making these characteristics and capabilities explicit, it is hoped that the future of social work in integrated mental health teams will be placed on a more secure footing.

The distinctive contribution of social work to interdisciplinary working in mental health

Social Work Perspectives and Knowledge Base

Social work is about change. Social workers try to improve the circumstances of people who are vulnerable or face social exclusion both by building on their personal strengths and by changing the social circumstances which have contributed to their mental distress. This means that they take a community as well as an individual perspective. They are committed to principles of self-determination and of helping people to overcome discrimination and other barriers to achieving their potential.

The social work knowledge base brings together a range of social science perspectives, linked to an understanding of law and social policy as it affects users of social care services and their families or informal carers. Seeing the person in their social context, practitioners apply social models of mental health, with an emphasis on how personal and family relationships, cultural needs, housing, work and social networks may be integral to recovery.

Social work has particular expertise in relation to the social and environmental factors that contribute to mental distress through the life course. This includes the impact of abuse and the impact of stigma on personal development.

The profession is characterised by a strong tradition of critical questioning, reflection and challenge within a multi-disciplinary context.

Essential Shared Capabilities

Social work has long provided a key and integral contribution to mental health services. Social work values, skills and knowledge are closely aligned with the 'Ten Essential Shared Capabilities' Framework for mental health practice and emphasise empowerment, challenging inequalities and working in partnership with service users and carers to support recovery.

Distinctive Practice Capabilities of Social Workers

- Assessing complex situations, taking account of an individual's strengths, aspirations, and vulnerabilities within a context of their personal and family relationships, cultural needs, social and environmental stressors and connections within the community.
- Working alongside service users to promote their social inclusion – mobilising a range of community resources, networks, and statutory and voluntary services.
- Balancing legal and human rights and issues of risk and safety – achieving the least restrictive alternative within statutory roles and responsibilities, while offering protection to those who may be at risk of exploitation or harm.

(Continued)

- Working with family and informal carers to support an individual's journey to recovery
- Identifying and working with the personal and social consequences of discrimination, stigma and abuse
- Seeking changes in the social and environmental context which will promote recovery

(NWW4SW Sub Group, in SWAP/MHHE, 2007: 10)

WHAT DO SERVICE USERS AND CARERS WANT FROM INTEGRATED MENTAL HEALTH TEAMS?

The subject of integration in mental health policy and practice has tended to be dominated by the voices and perspectives of government, academics and professionals (SPN, 2004). However, the case for the distinctive contribution of social workers in integrated mental health teams is supported by user and carer-centred research evidence that demonstrates the high value placed on the particular role that social workers play in assisting recovery. 'People who use services value the non-stigmatising help and access to services provided by social workers and the core values of social work practice directly support the independent living movement' (SCIE, 2008: 4).

The value of social workers for people with mental health problems – a service user perspective

Mental health isn't simply a medical issue; it's about how we function in the world and how we relate to others. Those of us with mental health problems have the same basic needs as other members of society, such as housing, finance, education, employment and family life. Social workers have the specialist skills to help and advise us in our efforts to meet these needs, all of which are important in maintaining good mental health and a role as an equal member of society.

So what do social workers offer?

Housing – knowledge of local accommodation, pricing structures and bureaucratic requirements, e.g. are pets allowed?
Benefits system – trained in welfare rights and can assist with benefit claims.
Education and employment – awareness of local resources and can encourage and support people in accessing education, from basic literacy skills to training for jobs, and in employment, both paid and voluntary.
Legal rights – trained in many legal aspects which are useful in child protection situations, court liaison work, disability discrimination, the Mental Health Act and much more.

Advocacy – knowledge of the law, welfare rights and tenancy rights enables social workers to advocate for clients.
Community – linking clients into statutory, private and voluntary services in the community, such as family centres, parent and toddler groups, social groups, creative activity groups or sports.

Social workers work alongside those of us with mental health problems to help us maintain our independence and support us on our road to recovery.

(cited in Foster, 2005: 5)

The value of social workers for carers of people with mental health problems – a carer perspective

Caring for loved ones who have enduring mental health problems often has major negative repercussions on the life of the carer:

- Mental and physical health
- Relationships with family and friends
- Ability to work and finances

Consequently, carers can have a great need for information, services and support. Social workers are uniquely qualified and best placed to help. Social workers think and see 'beyond taking tablets' to use the whole context for the carer (and service user) to bring about the best outcomes:

- Encouraging the carer to get support and respite (if needed)
- Assessing the needs of the carer and seeing through the implementation of the carer's care plan
- Assisting access to services and carers' grants
- Explaining pertinent aspects of the NSF 6 'Caring for Carers' and the 'Carers' Rights Act'

Social workers enhance best outcomes by listening to carers who have an important story to tell (albeit many times an extremely emotional one). Social workers can help channel this experience in positive directions in a way which medical staff or family and friends cannot. Most positively, social workers know that carers (and service users) are likely to be 'experts by experience' and will take advantage of their knowledge.

In that context, social workers play a key role in facing and balancing the sensitive issue of confidentiality. On the one hand, social workers supply carers with necessary non-confidential information. On the other, social workers actively encourage service users to understand the benefits of disclosing to others and engage service users to do so when appropriate.

(cited in Foster, 2005: 5)

Davis notes how the growing body of research evidence based on the experiences of people who use services and their carers gives a strong indication about the direction that integration should take (cited in SPN, 2004). This evidence not only highlights the priorities and service designs that should be driving integration but also points to the vital importance of the values that need to be embraced across the mental health workforce if integration is to make a positive difference to service users' and carers' lives. A key message is that integration is not just about providing a seamless service; it is about working with people who use services and carers in ways that build respect, understanding, self esteem and confidence in service users as well as workers. Davis suggests that in developing integrated mental health services the traditional psychiatrically driven service priorities need to be widened to accommodate a focus on the totality and complexity of individual's lives. She argues:

> This is more than a matter of health accommodating social care interests. It is a matter of health and social care professionals and researchers recognising that service user experience and expertise needs to be acknowledged and actively worked with in delivering on the integration agenda set by government .... Regardless of professional designation it is professionals who treat service users with respect, listen to what they are saying and work with them over time in relationships built on trust and mutual regard on priorities that make a positive contribution to service users realising their aspirations and an improved quality of life. (cited in SPN, 2004: 25)

A research project in Birmingham (designed by service users to gather data about how people who live with mental health problems experienced the mental health system) explored how jointly provided services might achieve better outcomes for service users. The main findings were that:

- Service users expected that contact with services would assist them in managing their mental health problems/diagnosed mental illness through times of crisis and recovery.
- Some services were experienced as hindering people to pursue their lives, aspirations and recovery. These were services in which people found they were treated as passive recipients, offered little information about what was on offer and few opportunities for exchanges with staff about their hopes and fears for the future.
- Some services were experienced as supporting people to pursue their lives and aspirations. These were services that valued people as experts on their own lives, connected with them as individuals and worked with them to transform their lives and support recovery.

The services that were valued by users provided:

- Opportunities for users on an individual and group basis to talk about their hopes, fears and aspirations for the future.
- Information about issues and concerns of importance in users' lives e.g. medication, life changes, treatment options, relationships, income, housing, employment, education.
- Advocacy in relation to key life areas as well as access to and exit from services.
- Relationships with staff and other users based on respect, mutual valuing and growing trust.

(Davis and Braithwaite, cited in SPN, 2004: 26)

Research findings such as these demonstrate how important it is for professionals to establish common values and goals for services that are consistent with what service users value. As Davis concludes, 'it is important that work on delivering integration is based on this evidence and rooted in what is happening and what could happen if services and professionals open up their current agendas so that service users are actively involved as partners. It is by working in this way from the bottom up that we will have a chance to make integration work for those who turn to mental health services for support' (cited in SPN, 2004: 27–28).

CHAPTER SUMMARY

In the space of a decade the organization and practice of social work has been transformed. The modern mental health system is driven by the development of new approaches, new specialisms and draws on the integrated skills of a variety of professionals. Social workers are now employed in a diverse range of contexts in the statutory, private, voluntary and independent sectors, many within integrated teams. At the very least they are expected to know how to work collaboratively and effectively with other professionals to provide services to users and carers. Meanwhile, the messages from users of mental health services and their carers are clear – regardless of their professional designation, *all* mental health professionals must be prepared to adapt their practice to meet the needs of users and carers.

Further reading/resources

Bogg, D. (2008) *The Integration of Mental Health Social Work and the NHS*. Exeter: Learning Matters.

Social Perspectives Network (2004) *SPN Paper 6. Integration of Health and Social Care: Promoting Social Care Perspectives within Integrated Mental Health Services*. London: Social Perspectives Network.

www.caipe.org.uk – Centre for the Advancement of Interprofessional Education.

CONCLUSION

In 2009 the National Service Framework for Mental Health – the policy framework underpinning mental health care in the UK for a decade – will come to an end. Inevitably it is a time for reflection on what has been achieved, what could or should have been achieved and where mental health policy and practice should go in the future. As we have outlined in this book, over the last decade the organization and structure of the mental health system has changed fundamentally and this has posed (and continues to pose) significant challenges for all mental health practitioners. But what of the impact of the changes on users of mental health services and their carers? In some respects it cannot be disputed that some of the changes have been positive. The profile of mental health has been raised; significant resources have been invested in mental health care and we have seen some imaginative innovations in models of service delivery. However, as with many other initiatives in mental health care that have preceded it, the NSFMH has still fallen short of its promises and some of its recommendations sadly remain rhetoric rather than reality.

In this book we have presented evidence that clearly demonstrates the persistence of inequalities in accessing the mental health system and of social exclusion and poor life outcomes for the mentally distressed. Currently mental health services do not adequately meet the needs of some people, while too many others (especially Black people) are over represented at the 'sharp end' of the system in detention and compulsion. These shortcomings 'are reflected in the consistently high levels of dissatisfaction from service users and other stakeholders about the national variability in standards of care and support' (Future Vision Coalition, 2008: 4).

At the beginning of the book we made the case for a critical social scientific approach to understanding the mental health system. It is often a misconception that 'being critical' equates with being negative. This is simply not true. Rather, critical social science exposes issues that would otherwise remain uncovered and uncontested. It challenges taken-for-granted ways of understanding the world, including ourselves. In the mental health context it enables us to see that, regardless of the assumed benevolent intentions of policy makers or mental health practitioners, users of mental health services can and do still experience the mental heath system as oppressive. Moreover, it enables us to see how their experiences of marginalization and exclusion are inextricably linked to the stigma of mental distress – a process in which the mental health system itself and the professionals within it are deeply implicated. While our historical analysis demonstrated that the mentally distressed have always been dehumanized, stigmatized and socially excluded, we have also seen how the medical model of mental health has reconstructed and perpetuated their status as 'other'. This message poses a fundamental challenge to all those who work in the mental health field. While mental health practice is entrenched in the traditions of the medical model of mental health we will fundamentally fail those in mental distress.

A critical social scientific approach to understanding mental health theory, law, policy and practice opens the door to new ways of looking at, making sense of and responding to people in mental distress. Moving forward means dealing with the messy contradictions inherent in relationships between professionals, users and carers, the public and the state. In this book we have challenged students of mental health to consider what it means to become a critically reflective mental health practitioner and readers should by now be under no illusion that it is an easy task. Being a critically reflective practitioner in the modern mental health system is risky and uncomfortable. It is not a technique or competency to be acquired. It is rooted in who we are and what we stand for (values) and is therefore essentially a *political* activity. It means setting one's face squarely against the tide of authoritarian populism and managerial pragmatism and speaking out against hypocrisy, injustice and oppression where we find it. It means refusing to accept that 'this is just the way things are', imagining how things could be and determining to be a part of a better system. It involves asking awkward questions and challenging assumptions at every turn. Of course this has consequences – both personally and professionally. It is exhausting, at times demoralizing and can often feel futile when two steps back follow each step forward.

We would argue that these are the enduring characteristics of mental health social work in particular and this is why it is essential that the profession must fight to retain its identity in the face of ongoing organizational change:

> Traditional expectations from social work itself have been to empower service users and carers through a range of value-based and evidence-based interventions within a social model and understanding of mental distress. The 'social' element in our culture (and title) has often been interpreted and polarised by some as assisting people with housing, financial and childcare issues. For others, social workers are seen as non-conforming, interfering politically correct risk-takers. Added to this is the 'necessary nuisance' a social care perspective brings to a service culturally dominated by the medical model, and which is particularly evident in the statutory framework. (CSIP/NIMHE, 2005: 14)

In its research briefing on *Mental Health and Social Work*, SCIE notes how 'analysis of the "essential capabilities" required for mental health practice emphasizes the centrality of a professional value base that promotes dignity, human worth and social justice and a commitment to the social perspectives of the recovery model' (2008: 4). Research on the practice of mental health social workers has demonstrated how their practice is entirely consistent with these expectations (DH/CSIP/NSIP, 2007). The other key messages from the research briefing (SCIE, 2008: 1) are:

- The traditional skills of social work remain important and social workers have a distinctive role in multi-agency settings.
- Social work needs to develop practices which help people with mental health problems identify and realize their own needs.
- Social work has a significant role to play in coordinating efforts to support individuals and groups who may often have negative experiences and perceptions of mental health services.

- Social workers need to maintain a broad social view of mental health problems especially in regard to concerns about discriminatory practices, civil rights and social justice.
- Policy makers need to focus on the role that social work plays in integrated mental health services and support further professional development.

The research briefing also stresses the importance of:

- Holistic approaches combining practical and emotional support.
- Reducing isolation and developing supportive networks.
- Promoting independence and self-directed support.

The Future Vision Coalition (2008: 4–5) has published a discussion paper on the future direction of mental health services in which it argues that all future policy relating to mental health must have three central aims:

1. To remove barriers to social inclusion – in particular, stigmatizing public attitudes and discriminatory behaviour – for all those experiencing and recovering from mental health problems.
2. To improve the life outcomes of those experiencing and recovering from mental health problems.
3. To improve the overall levels of mental health in the population.

In order to achieve these aims, it suggests that four fundamental policy changes are required:

1. A shift from the current medical model of mental health to an integrated model, where policy takes into account the impact of social and economic circumstances on mental health alongside individual psychological factors.
2. A positive approach to the mental well-being of the whole population through improving public understanding, creating conditions conducive to good mental health, increasing early recognition of problems, and preventing escalation of problems to crisis point.
3. For those who need support beyond that of family and friends, a change in focus away from simply reducing symptoms and towards enhancing their quality of life and supporting them to fulfil their ambitions.
4. Ensuring that the individual wanting support has the right to determine how and when that support is delivered, and is involved in its design, with the support of carers, family and community.

We would argue that the contribution of social work knowledge, skills and values are integral to this 'future vision' for mental health services. However, whether this will be realized remains to be seen.

Finally we hope that this book has succeeded in conveying our central message that if the mental health system is to change for the better then it needs to pay much closer attention to users of mental health services as 'experts by experience'. This means policy-makers and practitioners must listen to, respect and privilege the voices of the mentally distressed in mental health research and learn directly from them what works in promoting their recovery.

BIBLIOGRAPHY

Aldridge, J. and Becker, S. (2003) *Children Caring for Parents with Mental Illness: Perspectives of Young Carers, Parents and Professionals*. Bristol: The Policy Press.

Allcock, J. (2003) *Mental Health Services – Workforce Design and Development. Best Practice Guidance*. London: Department of Health.

American Psychiatric Association (2000) *Diagnostic and Statistical Manual of Mental Disorders*, 5th edn. DSM-IV-TR. Washington, DC: APA.

Angermeyer, M.C. and Matschinger, H. (2003) 'The stigma of mental illness: effects of labelling on public attitudes towards people with mental disorder', *Acta Psychiatrica Scandinavica*, 108(4): 304–9.

Arksey, H., O'Malley, L., Baldwin, S., Harris, J., Newbronner, E., Hare, P. and Mason, A. (2002) *Services to Support Carers of People with Mental Health Problems: an Overview Report*. York: Social Policy Research Unit, University of York.

Audit Commission (1986) *Making a Reality of Community Care*. London: HMSO.

Audit Commission (2003) *Human Rights: Improving Public Service Delivery*. London: Audit Commission.

Audit Commission (2005) *Governing Partnerships: Bridging the Accountability Gap*. London: Audit Commission.

Baker, S. and MacPherson, J. (2000) *Counting the Cost. Mental Health in the Media*. London: MIND.

Bamber, C. (2004) 'From grassroots to statute. The mental health service user movement in England', in T. Ryan and J. Pritchard (eds), *Good Practice in Adult Mental Health*. London: Jessica Kingsley Publishers.

Bamford, T. (2006) 'Social workers should play key role in mental health', *Community Care Magazine*, 6 July 2006, http://www.communitycare.co.uk/Articles/2006/07/06/54848/social-workers-should-play-key-role-in-mental-health.html

Barclay, P. (1982) *Social Workers: Their Role and Tasks*. London: NISW.

Barham, P. (1992) *Closing the Asylum. The Mental Health Patient in Modern Society*. London: Penguin.

Barn, R. (2008) 'Ethnicity, gender and mental health: social worker perspectives', *International Journal of Social Psychiatry*, 54(1): 69–82.

Barnes, M. and Bowl, R. (2001) *Taking Over the Asylum: Empowerment and Mental Health*. Basingstoke: Palgrave.

Barr, H. and Ross, F. (2006) 'Mainstreaming interprofessional education in the United Kingdom: a position paper', *Journal of Interprofessional Care*, 20(2): 96–104.

Bartlett, P. and Wright, D. (eds) (1999) *Outside the Walls of the Asylum: The History of Care in the Community 1750–2000*. London: Athlone Press.

BASW (British Association of Social Workers) (2002) *Code of Ethics for Social Work*. Birmingham: British Association of Social Workers.

Bebbington, P., Targosz, S. and Lewis, G. (2002) *Lone Mothers, Social Exclusion and Depression*. London: Royal College of Psychiatrists Annual Conference.

Beckett, C. and Maynard, A. (2005) *Values and Ethics in Social Work. An Introduction*. London: Sage.

Bentall, R. (2004) *Madness Explained: Psychosis and Human Nature*. London: Allen Lane.

Beresford, P. (2007a) 'User involvement, research and health inequalities: developing new directions', *Health and Social Care in the Community*, 15(4): 306–12.

Beresford, P. (2007b) *The Changing Roles and Tasks of Social Work From Service User Perspectives. A Literature Informed Discussion Paper*. London: Shaping Our Lives.

Beresford, P. (2008) *Making Personalisation Work, 2nd SPN Personalisation Conference*, 8 December 2008, http://www.spn.org.uk/fileadmin/SPN_uploads/Documents/PB Personalisation.doc (accessed 19 December 2008).

Berzins, K.M., Petch, A. and Atkinson, J.M. (2003) 'Prevalence and experience of harassment of people with mental health problems living in the community', *British Journal of Psychiatry*, 183: 526–33.

Black, N. (2001) 'Evidence based policy: proceed with care', *British Medical Journal*, 323: 275–8.

Blaxter, M. (1990) *Health and Lifestyles*. London: Routledge.

Boardman, J. (2005) 'New services for old – an overview of mental health policy', in Sainsbury Centre for Mental Health, *Beyond the Water Towers: The Unfinished Revolution in Mental Health Services 1985–2005*. London: Sainsbury Centre for Mental Health.

Bogg, D. (2007) 'An injection of social care', *Community Care Magazine*, 29 March.

Bornat, J., Johnson, J., Pereira, C., Pilgrim, D. and Williams, F. (1997) *Community Care: A Reader*, 2nd edn. Buckingham: Open University Press.

Borrill, C.S., Carletta, J., Carter, A.J., Dawson, J.F., Garrod, S., Rees, A., Richards, A., Shapiro, D. and West, M.A. (2000) *The Effectiveness of Healthcare Teams in the National Health Service*. Birmingham: Aston University.

Bracken, P. (2002) 'Depression, psychiatry and the use of ECT', *Asylum Magazine*, 12(4): 26–8.

Bracken, P. and Smyth, M. (2006) 'Rebalancing the approach to mental health', *Irish Times*, 29 December 2006.

Bracken, P. and Thomas, P. (2000) 'Putting ethics before effectiveness', *Open Mind*, 102: 22.

Brammer, A. (2007) *Social Work Law*, 2nd edn. Harlow: Pearson/Longman.

Breggin, P. (2008) *Brain-Disabling Treatments in Psychiatry*. New York: Springer Publishing Company.

Brewis, R. (2008) *A New Hope?* http://www.spn.org.uk/fileadmin/SPN_uploads/Documents/rb_personalisation.pdf (accessed 3 June 2008).

British Institute of Human Rights (2002) *Something for Everyone*. London: British Institute of Human Rights.

Broverman, I.K., Broverman, D.M., Clarkson, F.E., Rosenkrantz, P.S. and Volgel, S.R. (1970) 'Sex role stereotypes and clinical judgement of mental health', *Journal of Consulting and Clinical Psychology*, 34, 1–7.

Brown, P. (1985) *Mental Health Care and Social Policy*. London: RKP.

Brown, G.W. and Harris, T. (1978) *Social Origins of Depression: A Study of Psychiatric Disorders in Women*. London: Tavistock.

Burman, E. (1994) *Deconstructing Developmental Psychology*. London: Routledge.

Busfield, J. (1986) *Managing Madness: Changing Ideas and Practice*. London: Hutchinson.

Bynum, W.F., Porter, R. and Shepherd, M. (1985) *The Anatomy of Madness*. London: Tavistock.

Bytheway, B. (1995) *Ageism*. Buckingham: Open University Press.

Campbell, P. (2005) 'From little acorns – the mental health service user movement', in Sainsbury Centre for Mental Health, *Beyond the Water Towers: The Unfinished Revolution in Mental Health Services 1985–2005*. London: Sainsbury Centre for Mental Health.

Carr, S. (2003) 'Lesbian and gay perspectives on mental distress', in Social Perspectives Network, *SPN Paper 3. Start Making Sense ... Developing Social Models to Understand and Work with Mental Distress*. London: Social Perspectives Network.

Chaplin, R. (2000) 'Psychiatrists can cause stigma too', *British Journal of Psychiatry*, 177: 467.
Chesler, P. (1972) *Women and Madness*. New York: Doubleday.
Citizen's Advice Bureau (2004) *Out of the Picture: CAB Evidence on Mental Health and Social Exclusion*. London: Citizen's Advice Bureau.
Clarke, J. (ed.) (1993) *A Crisis in Care?* London: Sage/Open University.
Clarke, J. (2004) 'Mad, bad and dangerous: the media and mental illness', *Mental Health Practice*, 7(10): 16–19.
Clements, J. (1998) 'A third way for mental illness?', *Community Care Magazine*, 1252: 16–22.
Cobb, A. (1993) *Safe and Effective? MIND's Views on Psychiatric Drugs, ECT and Psychosurgery*. London: MIND.
Cochrane, A. (1993) 'Challenges from the centre', in J. Clarke (ed.), *A Crisis in Care?* London: Sage/Open University.
Coleman, R. (1999) *Recovery: An Alien Concept*. Gloucester: Handsell Publishing.
Commission for Healthcare Audit and Inspection (2005) *Count Me In, Results of a National Census of Inpatients in Mental Health Hospitals and Facilities in England and Wales*. London: Commission for Healthcare, Audit and Inspection.
Cook, G., Gerrish, K. and Clarke, C. (2001) 'Decision-making in teams: issues arising from two UK evaluations', *Journal of Interprofessional Care*, 15(2): 141–51.
Coppock, V. (1997) 'Mad, bad or misunderstood?', in P. Scraton (ed.), *'Childhood' in 'Crisis'*. London: UCL Press.
Coppock, V. (2002) 'Medicalising children's behaviour' in B. Franklin (ed.), *The New Handbook of Children's Rights: Comparative Policy and Practice*, 2nd edn. London: Routledge.
Coppock, V. (2005) 'Mad, bad or misunderstood?' Revised and updated, in H. Hendrick (ed.), *Child Welfare and Social Policy: an Essential Reader*. London: The Policy Press.
Coppock, V. (2008) 'Gender', in R. Tummey and T. Turner (eds), *Critical Issues in Mental Health*. Basingstoke: Palgrave Macmillan.
Coppock, V. and Hopton, J. (2000) *Critical Perspectives on Mental Health*. London: Routledge.
Crossley, N. (1999) 'Fish, field, habitus and madness: the first wave mental health users movement in Britain', *British Journal of Sociology*, 50(4): 647–70.
CSCI (Commission for Social Care Inspection) and the Healthcare Commission (2007) *No Voice, No Choice. A Joint Review of Adult Community Mental Health Services in England*. London: Commission for Healthcare, Audit and Inspection.
CSIP (Care Services Improvement Partnership) and NIMHE (National Institute for Mental Health in England) (in collaboration with Association of Directors of Social Services, British Association of Social Workers, Department of Health, General Social Care Council, Social Care Institute for Excellence, Skills for Care and Social Perspectives Network) (2005) *The Social Work Contribution to Mental Health Services. The Future Direction. A Discussion Paper*. Leeds: NIMHE.
CSIP (Care Services Improvement Partnership) and NIMHE (National Institute for Mental Health in England) (2008) *Three Keys to a Shared Approach in Mental Health Assessment*. London: DH.
CSIP (Care Services Improvement Partnership), RCPsych (Royal College of Psychiatrists) and SCIE (Social Care Institute for Excellence) (2007) *A Common Purpose: Recovery in Future Mental Health Services*. London: Social Care Institute for Excellence.
CSIP (Care Services Improvement Partnership) and Shift (2006) *Mind Over Matter. Improving Media Reporting of Mental Health*. London: CSIP/Shift.
Danbury, H. (1976) 'Mental health compulsory admissions', *Social Work Today*, 7(6): 172–4.
Davies, M. (1981) *The Essential Social Worker*, 1st edn. Aldershot: Ashgate.
DCSF (Department for Children, Schools and Families) (2007) *The Children's Plan: Building Brighter Futures*. London: HMSO.

De Swaan, A. (1990) *The Management of Normality*. London: Routledge.
Department for Work and Pensions (2002) *Disabled for Life*. London: DWP.
DH (Department of Health) (1989) *Caring for People: Community Care in the Next Decade and Beyond*. London: HMSO.
DH (Department of Health) (1990) *Community Care in the Next Decade and Beyond. Policy Guidance*. London: HMSO.
DH (Department of Health) (1995) *Building Bridges: A Guide to Arrangements for Inter-Agency Working for the Care and Protection of Severely Mentally Ill People*. London: DH.
DH (Department of Health) (1997) *The New NHS: Modern, Dependable*. London: DH.
DH (Department of Health) (1998a) *Modernising Mental Health Services: Safe, Sound and Supportive*. London: DH.
DH (Department of Health) (1998b) *Partnership in Action: New Opportunities for Joint Working Between Health and Social Services – A Discussion Document*. London: DH.
DH (Department of Health) (1999a) *The National Service Framework for Mental Health. Modern Standards and Service Models*. London: DH.
DH (Department of Health) (1999b) *Effective Care Co-ordination: Modernising the Care Programme Approach*. London: DH.
DH (Department of Health) (2000) *The NHS Plan. A Plan for Investment, a Plan for Reform*. London: DH.
DH (Department of Health) (2001a) *The Mental Health Policy Implementation Guide*. London: DH.
DH (Department of Health) (2001b) *Shifting the Balance of Power*. London: DH.
DH (Department of Health) (2002a) *Shifting the Balance of Power: the Next Steps*. London: DH.
DH (Department of Health) (2002b) *Women's Mental Health: Into the Mainstream – Strategic Development of Mental Health Care for Women*. London: DH.
DH (Department of Health) (2002c) *National Suicide Prevention Strategy for England*. London: DH.
DH (Department of Health) (2003a) *Attitudes to Mental Illness*. London: DH.
DH (Department of Health) (2003b) *Electro-convulsive Therapy: Survey Covering the Period from January 2002 to March 2002, England. Statistical Bulletin 2003/08*. London: DH.
DH (Department of Health) (2003c) *Mainstreaming Gender and Women's Mental Health: Implementation Guidance*. London: DH.
DH (Department of Health) (2003d) *Every Child Matters*. London: DH.
DH (Department of Health) (2004) *The Ten Essential Shared Capabilities: A Framework for the Whole of the Mental Health Workforce*. London: DH.
DH (Department of Health) (2005a) *Your Care, Your Say. Public Consultation*. London: HMSO.
DH (Department of Health) (2005b) *Independence, Well-being and Choice: Our Vision for the Future of Adult Social Care for Adults in England*. London: DH.
DH (Department of Health) (2005c) *Delivering Race Equality in Mental Health Care: An Action Plan for Reform Inside and Outside Services and the Government's Response to the Independent Inquiry into the Death of David Bennett*. London: DH.
DH (Department of Health) (2005d) *New Ways of Working for Psychiatrists: Enhancing Effective, Person-Centred Services through New Ways of Working in Multidisciplinary and Multi-agency Contexts: Final Report 'But Not the End of the Story'*. London: DH.
DH (Department of Health) (2006) *Our Health, Our Care, Our Say: a New Direction for Community Services*. London: DH.
DH (Department of Health) (2007a) *Putting People First: a Shared Vision and Commitment to the Transformation of Adult Social Care*. London: DH.
DH (Department of Health) (2007b) *Best Practice in Managing Risk: Principles and Evidence for Best Practice in the Assessment and Management of Risk to Self and Others in Mental Health Services*. London: DH.

DH (Department of Health) (2007c) *New Ways of Working in Mental Health*. London: DH.
DH (Department of Health) (2007d) *Creating an Interprofessional Workforce: an Education and Training Framework for the Health and Social Care Workforce in England*. London: DH.
DH (Department of Health) (2007e) *New Ways of Working for Everyone. Developing and Sustaining a Capable and Flexible Workforce. Progress Report*. London: DH.
DH (Department of Health) (2007f) *Creating Capable Teams Approach. New Ways of Working in Mental Health*. London: DH.
DH (Department of Health) (2008a) *Carers at the Heart of 21st Century Families and Communities: a Caring System On Your Side, a Life of Your Own*. London: DH.
DH (Department of Health) (2008b) *Refocusing the Care Programme Approach: Policy and Positive Practice Guidance*. London: DH.
DH (Department of Health) (2008c) *Transforming Social Care*. London: DH. http://www.dh.gov.uk/en/Publicationsandstatistics/Lettersandcirculars/LocalAuthorityCirculars/DH_081934 (accessed 19 December 2008).
DH (Department of Health) (2008d) *Personalisation*, http://www.dh.gov.uk/en/SocialCare/Socialcarereform/Personalisation/index.htm (accessed 19 December 2008).
DH (Department of Health) (2008e) *Reference Guide to the Mental Health Act 1983*. London: TSO.
DH (Department of Health) (2008f) *Code of Practice: Mental Health Act 1983 (revised May 2008)*. London: TSO.
DH (Department of Health) (2008g) *Human Rights in Healthcare: a Framework for Local Action*, 2nd edn. London: DH.
DH (Department of Health), CSIP (Care Services Improvement Partnership) and NSIP (National Social Inclusion Programme) (2007) *Capabilities for Inclusive Practice*. London: DH.
DHSS (Department of Health and Social Security) (1975) *Better Services for the Mentally Ill*. London: DHSS.
Disability Rights Commission (2007) *Coming Together: Mental Health, Equality and Human Rights*. London: DRC.
Donnelly, M. (1983) *Managing the Mind*. London: Tavistock.
Donzelot, J. (1980) *The Policing of Families*. London: Hutchinson.
Double, D.B. (2001) 'The overemphasis on biomedical diagnosis in psychiatry', *Journal of Critical Psychology, Counselling and Psychotherapy*, 2: 40–7.
Double, D.B. (2002) 'The limits of psychiatry', *British Medical Journal*, 324: 900–4.
Doyal, L. (2000) *Health and Work in Older Women: a Neglected Issue*. London: The Pennell Initiative for Women's Health.
Driver, F. (1993) *Power and Pauperism*. Cambridge: Cambridge University Press.
DTI (Department of Trade and Industry) (2005) *Public Sector Duty to Promote Gender Equality*. London: DTI.
Duggan, M., Cooper, A. and Foster, J. (2002) *Modernising the Social Model in Mental Health: A Discussion Paper*. London: Social Perspectives Network/TOPSS England.
Dunn, S. (1999) *Creating Accepting Communities: Report of the Mind Inquiry into Social Exclusion and Mental Health Problems*. London: MIND.
Dustin, D. (2007) *The McDonaldisation of Social Work*. London: Ashgate.
Engels, F. (1973) *The Condition of the Working Class in England*. London: Lawrence & Wishart.
Equality and Human Rights Commission (2008) 'Public authorities and human rights', http://www.equalityhumanrights.com/en/forbusinessesandorganisation/publicauthorities/Pages/HumanRights.aspx (accessed 23 November 2008).
Faulkner, A. (1997) *Knowing Our Own Minds*. London: Mental Health Foundation.
Faulkner, A. and Layzell, S. (2000) *Strategies for Living: A Report of User-Led Research into People's Strategies for Living with Mental Distress*. London: Mental Health Foundation.

Faulkner, A. and Thomas, P. (2002) 'User-led Research and Evidence-Based Medicine', *British Journal of Psychiatry*, 180: 1–3.
Fennell, P. (1996) *Treatment Without Consent*. London: Routledge.
Fernando, S. (1995) *Mental Health in a Multi-ethnic Society*. London: Routledge.
Fernando, S. (2002) *Mental Health, Race and Culture*, 2nd edn. Basingstoke: Palgrave Macmillan.
Fernando, S. (2003) *Cultural Diversity, Mental Health and Psychiatry: the Struggle Against Racism*. London: Brunner Routledge.
Fernando, S. (2008) 'Institutional racism and cultural diversity', in R. Tummey and T. Turner (eds), *Critical Issues in Mental Health*. Basingstoke: Palgrave Macmillan.
Finch, J. and Groves, D. (1983) *A Labour of Love: Women, Work and Caring*. London: RKP.
Fook, J. (2007) 'Uncertainty: the defining characteristic of social work?', in M. Lymbery and K. Postle (eds), *Social Work*. London: Sage.
Foster, J. (2005) *Where Are We Going? The Social Work Contribution to Mental Health Services. A Discussion Paper Drafted on Behalf of and with Contributions from SCIE, NIMHE, GSCC, Skills for Care, ADSS, BASW, DH*. London: Social Perspectives Network.
Foucault, M. (1967) *Madness and Civilisation*. London: Tavistock.
Foucault, M. (1977) *Discipline and Punish: The Birth of the Prison*. London: Allen Lane.
Foucault, M. (1979) 'On governmentality', *Ideology and Consciousness*, 6: 5–21.
Francis, E. (1996) 'Community care, danger and black people', *Openmind*, 80: 4–5.
Frosh, S. (1997) 'Screaming under the bridge: masculinity, rationality and psychotherapy', in J.M. Ussher (ed.), *Body Talk: The Material and Discursive Regulation of Sexuality, Madness and Reproduction*. London: Routledge.
Future Vision Coalition (2008) *A New Vision for Mental Health. Discussion Paper*, http://www.newvisionformentalhealth.org.uk/index.html
General Social Care Council (2002) *Code of Practice for Social Care Workers*. London: General Social Care Council.
Gibbons, J. (1988) 'Residential care for mentally ill adults', in I. Sinclair (ed.), *Residential Care: The Research Reviewed*. London: HMSO.
Gilbert, P. (2003) *The Value of Everything: Social Work and its Importance in the Field of Mental Health*. Lyme Regis: Russell House Publishing.
Glendinning, C. and Arksey, H. (2008) 'Informal care', in P. Alcock, M. May and K. Rowlingson (eds), *The Student's Companion to Social Policy*, 3rd edn. Oxford: Blackwell.
Goffman, E. (1961) *Asylums: Essays on the Social Situation of Mental Patients and Other Inmates*. Harmondsworth: Penguin.
Griffiths, Sir R. (1988) *Community Care: An Agenda for Action*. London: HMSO.
GSCC (General Social Care Council) (2002) *Codes of Practice for Social Care Workers and Employers*. London: General Social Care Council.
GSCC (General Social Care Council) (2008) *Roles and Tasks of Social Workers*. London: General Social Care Council.
Gulliver, P. (1999) 'Two approaches to the joint commissioning of mental health services', *Mental Health Review*, 4(3): 21–3.
Hannigan, B. (2003) 'The policy and legal context', in B. Hannigan and M. Coffey (eds), *The Handbook of Community Mental Health Nursing*. London: Routledge.
Harris, J. (2003) *The Social Work Business*. London: Routledge.
Harrison, G. (2002) 'Ethnic minorities and the Mental Health Act', *The British Journal of Psychiatry*, 180: 198–9.
Hawton, K. (1998) 'Why has suicide increased in young males?', *Crisis: Journal of Crisis Intervention and Suicide*, 19(3): 119–24.
Hawton, K. (2000) 'Sex and suicide: gender differences in suicidal behaviour', *British Journal of Psychiatry*, 177(6), 484–5.

Healthcare Commission, Mental Health Act Commission, National Institute for Mental Health in England (2005) *Count Me In: Results of a National Census of Inpatients in Mental Health Hospitals and Facilities in England and Wales*. London: Healthcare Commission.

Helm, A. (2003) 'Recovery and reclamation: a pilgrimage in understanding who and what we are', in P. Barker (ed.), *Psychiatric and Mental Health Nursing: The Craft of Caring*. London: Arnold.

Heyes, S. (2005) *Art of Recovery: a Pocket Guide to Recovering from Mental Illness*. South Somerset: MIND.

Hogman, G. and Pearson, G. (1995) *The Silent Partners: the Needs and Experiences of People who Provide Informal Care to People with a Severe Mental Illness*. Kingston upon Thames: National Schizophrenia Fellowship.

Hollingshead, A.B. and Redlich, F.C. (1958) *Social Class and Mental Illness: a Community Study*. New York: John Wiley.

Horner, N. (2003) *What is Social Work?* Exeter: Learning Matters.

Hudson, B. (2002) 'Integrated care and structural change in England: the case of Care Trusts', *Policy Studies*, 23(2): 77–95.

Humm, M. (1995) *The Dictionary of Feminist Theory*, 2nd edn. Hemel Hempstead: Prentice Hall/Harvester Wheatsheaf.

Hunt, R. and Fish, J. (2008) *Prescription for Change: Lesbian and Bisexual Women's Health Check 2008*. London: Stonewall.

Huxley, P., Evans, S., Gately, C., Webber, M., Mears, A., Pajak, S., Kendall, T., Medina, J. and Katona, C. (2005a) 'Stress and pressures in mental health social work: the worker speaks', *British Journal of Social Work*, 35: 1063–79.

Huxley, P., Evans, S., Webber, M. and Gately, C. (2005b) 'Staff shortages in the mental health workforce: the case of the disappearing approved social worker', *Health & Social Care in the Community*, 13(6): 504–13.

Integrated Care Network (2008) *A Practical Guide to Integrated Working*. London: Care Services Improvement Partnership/Integrated Care Network.

Irvine, E. (1978) 'Psychiatric social work', in E. Younghusband (ed.), *Social Work in Britain: 1950–1975*. London: Allen & Unwin.

Itzin, C. (2006) *Tackling the Health and Mental Health Effects of Domestic and Sexual Violence and Abuse*. London: Department of Health.

Jodelet, D. (1991) *Madness and Social Representations*. London: Harvester Wheatsheaf.

Johns, R. (2007) *Using the Law in Social Work*, 3rd edn. Exeter: Learning Matters.

Johnstone, L. (1999) 'Adverse psychological effects of ECT', *Journal of Mental Health*, 8(1): 69–85.

Jones, K. (1955) *Lunacy, Law and Conscience (1744–1845)*. London: RKP.

Jones, K. (1972) *A History of the Mental Health Services*. London: RKP.

Jones, K. (1993) *Asylums and After*. London: Athlone Press.

Jones, K., Brown, J. and Bradshaw, J. (1978) *Issues in Social Policy*. London: RKP.

Jones, C., Ferguson, I., Lavalette, M. and Penketh, L. (2004) *Social Work and Social Justice: a Manifesto for a New Engaged Practice*, http://www.liv.ac.uk/ssp/Social_Work_Manifesto.html (accessed 28 June 2008).

Jordan, B. (1997) 'Social work and society', in M. Davies (ed.), *The Blackwell Companion to Social Work*. London: Blackwell.

Kemshall, H. (2002) *Risk, Social Policy and Welfare*. Buckingham: Open University Press.

Kendall, T. (2006) *Some Systemic Problems in Translating Evidence into Clinical Practice: Case Studies from NICE Guidelines in Mental Health*. National Collaborating Centre for Mental Health, 9 June 2006, http://www.lse.ac.uk/collections/BIOS/pdf/rcts/Kendall.pdf (accessed 17 March 2008).

King, M. and McKeown, E. (2003) *Mental Health and Social Wellbeing of Gay Men, Lesbians and Bisexuals in England and Wales*. London: MIND.

King, M., Semlyen, J., See Tai, S., Killaspy, H., Osborn, D., Popelyuk, D. and Nazareth, I. (2007) *Mental Disorders, Suicide and Deliberate Self Harm in Lesbian, Gay and Bisexual People: a Systematic Review*. Leeds: NIMHE.

Kirk, H. and Kutchins, S. (1999) *Making Us Crazy: DSM: The Psychiatric Bible and the Creation of Mental Disorders*. London: Constable.

Kirsch, I., Deacon, B.J., Huedo-Medina, T.B., Scoboria, A., Moore, T.J. and Johnson, B.T. (2008) 'Initial severity and antidepressant benefits: a meta-analysis of data submitted to the Food and Drug Administration', *PLoS Medicine*, 5(2): e45, doi:10.1371/journal.pmed.0050045.

Laing, R.D. (1959) *The Divided Self*. London: Tavistock.

Laming, Lord (2003) *The Victoria Climbié Inquiry. Report of an Inquiry by Lord Laming*. London: HMSO.

Langan, M. (1993) 'The rise and fall of social work', in J. Clarke (ed.), *A Crisis in Care?* London: Sage/Open University.

Langan, J. and Means, R. (1995) *Personal Finances: Elderly People with Dementia and the 'New' Community Care*. London: Anchor Housing Trust.

Laurence, J. (2003) *Pure Madness: How Fear Drives the Mental Health System*. London: Routledge.

Le Grand, J. (1993) *Quasi-Markets and Social Policy*. Basingstoke: Palgrave.

Leason, K. (2004) 'Independence under fire', *Community Care Magazine*, 7–13 October, 30–1.

Lewis, J. and Glennerster, H. (1998) *Implementing the New Community Care*. Buckingham: Open University Press.

Loring, M. and Powell, B. (1988) 'Gender, race and DSMIII: a study of the objectivity of psychiatric diagnostic behaviour', *Journal of Health and Social Behaviour*, 29: 1–22.

Lupton, D. (1999) *Risk*. London: Routledge.

MacKenzie, C. (1992) *Psychiatry for the Rich*. London: Routledge.

Macpherson, Sir W. (1999) *The Stephen Lawrence Inquiry: Report of an Inquiry by Sir William Macpherson of Cluny*. London: HMSO.

Malek, M. (1991) *Psychiatric Admissions: A Report on Young People Entering Residential Psychiatric Care*. London: The Children's Society.

Mandelstam, M. (2005) *Community Care Practice and The Law*, 3rd edn. London: Jessica Kingsley Publishers.

Marshall, J.R. (1996) 'Science, "schizophrenia", and genetics: the creation of myths', *The Journal of Primary Prevention*, 17(1): 99–115.

Masson, J. (1990) *Against Therapy*. London: Fontana.

McCauley, J., Kern, D.E., Kolodner, K., Dill, L., Schroeder, A.F., DeChant, H.K., Ryden, J., Derogatis, L.R. and Bass, E.B. (1997) 'Clinical characteristics of women with a history of child abuse: unhealed wounds', *Journal of the American Medical Association*, 277: 1362–8.

McFarlane, L. (1998) *Diagnosis Homophobic: The Experiences of Lesbians, Gay Men and Bisexuals in Mental Health Services*. London: PACE.

McKay, D. (2000) 'Stigmatising pharmaceutical advertisements', *British Journal of Psychiatry*, 177: 467–8.

McKenna, H. (2003) 'Evidence-based practice in mental health care', in P. Barker (ed.), *Psychiatric and Mental Health Nursing: The Craft of Caring*. London: Arnold.

McKnight, J. (1995) *The Careless Society: Community and its Counterfeits*. New York: Basic Books.

McLaughlin, K. (2008) *Social Work, Politics and Society*. Bristol: The Policy Press.

Means, R. and Smith, R. (1998) *Community Care: Policy and Practice*, 2nd edn. London: Macmillan.

Meltzer, H., Gatwood, R., Goodman, R. and Ford, T. (2000) *Mental Health of Children and Adolescents in Great Britain*. London: The Stationery Office.

Meltzer, H. (1995) *OPCS Surveys of Psychiatric Morbidity in Great Britain: 1995*. London: HMSO.

MHAC (Mental Health Act Commission) (2004) *The Mental Health Act Commission's ECT Survey 1999–2002*. Nottingham: Mental Health Act Commission.

Mental Health Foundation (1998) *The Big Picture: Promoting Children and Young People's Mental Health*. London: Mental Health Foundation.

Mental Health Foundation (1999) *Bright Futures: Promoting Children and Young People's Mental Health*. London: Mental Health Foundation.

Mental Health Foundation (2000) *Pull Yourself Together! A Survey of the Stigma and Discrimination Faced by People who Experience Mental Distress*. London: Mental Health Foundation.

Mental Health Foundation (2002) *Out at Work: A Survey of the Experiences of People with Mental Health Problems within the Workplace*. London: Mental Health Foundation.

Mental Health Foundation (2003) Surviving User-Led Research: Reflections on Supporting User-Led Research Projects. London: Mental Health Foundation.

Mental Health Foundation, MIND, Rethink, Sainsbury Centre for Mental Health and Young Minds (2006) *We Need to Talk. The Case for Psychological Therapy on the NHS*. London: MIND.

Mental Health Media (2008) *Open Up. Mental Health Media's Anti-discrimination Toolkit*, http://www.openuptoolkit.net/discrimination_facts/discrimination_facts.php (accessed 1July 2008).

Millar, B. (2000) 'All in a day's work', *Therapy Weekly*, 27(10): 48.

Milne, A. and Williams, J. (2003) *Women in Transition – a Literature Review of the Mental Health Risks Facing Women in Mid-life*. London: The Pennell Initiative for Women's Health.

MIND (2001a) *MIND's Yellow Card for Reporting Drug Side Effects: A Report of Users' Experiences*. London: MIND.

MIND (2001b) *Roads to Recovery*. London: MIND.

MIND (2003a) *Factsheet. Public Attitudes to Mental Illness*. London: MIND.

MIND (2003b) *The Mental Health of the South Asian Community in Britain*. London: MIND. www.mind.org.uk/Information/Factsheets/Diversity/MHSACB.htm (accessed 15 June 2008).

MIND (2005) *Factsheet. Older People and Mental Health*. London: MIND. www.mind.org.uk/Information/Factsheets/Older+people/Older+People+and+Mental+Health.htm (accessed 28 October 2008).

MIND (2006) *Factsheet. The Mental Health of the African Caribbean community in Britain*. London: Mind. www.mind.org.uk/Information/Factsheets/Diversity/The+African+Caribbean+Community+and+Mental+Health.htm (accessed 15 June 2008).

MIND (2007a) *Public Attitudes to Mental Distress*. London: MIND. http://www.mind.org.uk/Information/Factsheets/Public+attitudes/

MIND (2007b) *Ecotherapy. The Green Agenda for Mental Health*. London: MIND.

MIND (2008a) *The Mental Health Act 1983. An Outline Guide*. London: MIND.

MIND (2008b) *Factsheet. Lesbians, Gay Men, Bisexuals and Mental Health*. London: MIND. www.mind.org.uk/Information/Factsheets/Diversity/Factsheetlgb.htm (accessed 27 October 2008).

Ministry of Justice (2008) *Human Rights Insight Project*. London: Ministry of Justice.

Monahan, J. (1992) 'Mental disorder and violent behaviour: attitudes and evidence', *American Psychologist*, 47: 511–21.

Moncrieff, J. (2003) 'Is psychiatry for sale? An examination of the influence of the pharmaceutical industry on academic and practical psychiatry', Maudsley Discussion Paper No. 13, Institute of Psychiatry, London. www.critpsynet.freeuk.com/pharmaceuticalindustry.htm

Moncrieff, J. (2006) 'Why is it so difficult to stop psychiatric drug treatment? It may be nothing to do with the original problem', *Medical Hypotheses*, 67(3): 517–23.

Morris, J. (2004a) *Services for People with Physical Impairments and Mental Health Support Needs*. York: Joseph Rowntree Foundation.

Morris, J. (2004b) *'One Town for my Body, Another for my Mind': Services for People with Physical Impairments and Mental Health Support Needs*. York: Joseph Rowntree Foundation.

Moving People (2008) *Stigma Shout. Service User and Carer Experiences of Stigma and Discrimination*. London: Moving People.

Muijen, M. (1995) 'Mental illness and crime', in *Community Care* (ed.), *Scare in the Community. Britain in a Moral Panic*. London: Reed Business Publishing.

Mullen, P., Martin, J., Anderson, J., Romans, S.E. and Herbison, P. (1993) 'Childhood sexual abuse and mental health in adult life', *British Journal of Psychiatry*, 163: 721–32.

Murphy, E. (1991) *After the Asylums: Community Care for People with Mental Illness*. London: Faber and Faber.

Murphy, E. (1982) 'Social origins of depression in old age', *British Journal of Psychiatry*, 141: 135–42.

NALGO (1989) *Social Work in Crisis: A Study in Six Local Authorities*. London: NALGO.

National Schizophrenia Fellowship Scotland (2001) *Give Us a Break: Exploring Harassment of People with Mental Health Problems*. Edinburgh: NSF Scotland.

National Steering Group (2004) *Guidance on New Ways of Working for Psychiatrists in a Multi-disciplinary and Multi-agency Context: Interim Report*. London: Department of Health.

Nazroo, J. and King, M. (2002) 'Psychosis – symptoms and estimated rates', in K. Sproston, and J. Nazroo (eds), *Ethnic Minority Psychiatric Illness Rates in the Community (Empiric)*. London: The Stationery Office.

Newnes, C. (1999) 'Histories of psychiatry', in C. Newnes, G. Holmes and C. Dunn (eds), *This is Madness: A Critical Look at Psychiatry and the Future of Mental Health Services*. Ross on Wye: PCCS Books.

Newnes, C. and Holmes, G. (1999) 'The future of mental health services', in C. Newnes, G. Holmes and C. Dunn (eds), *This is Madness: A Critical Look at Psychiatry and the Future of Mental Health Services*. Ross on Wye: PCCS Books.

NHS Management Executive (1994) *Introduction of Supervision Registers for Mentally Ill People from 1 April 1994 (HSG (94) 5)*. London: DH.

NICE (National Institute for Clinical Excellence) (2003) *Guidance on the Use of Electroconvulsive Therapy*. London: NICE.

NICE (National Institute for Clinical Excellence) (2007a) *Anxiety: NICE Clinical Guideline 22 (amended)*. London: NICE.

NICE (National Institute for Clinical Excellence) (2007b) *Depression: Management of Depression in Primary and Secondary Care. National Clinical Practice Guideline 23 (amended)*. London: NICE.

NIMHE (National Institute for Mental Health in England) (2003) *Inside Outside, Improving Mental Health Services for Black and Minority Ethnic Communities in England*. Leeds: NIMHE.

NIMHE (National Institute for Mental Health in England) (2005) *The Social Work Contribution to Mental Health Services: The Future Direction. A Discussion Paper*. Leeds: NIMHE.

NIMHE (National Institute for Mental Health in England) (2006) *The Social Work Contribution to Mental Health Services: The Future Direction. Report of Responses to the Discussion Paper*. Leeds: NIMHE.

Norfolk, Suffolk and Cambridgeshire Strategic Health Authority (2003) *Independent Inquiry into the Death of David Bennett*.

Norman, I.J. and Peck, E. (1999) 'Working together in adult community mental health services: an inter-professional dialogue', *Journal of Mental Health*, 8(3): 217–30.
Offe, C. (1984) *Contradictions of the Welfare State*. London: Hutchinson.
Office of the Deputy Prime Minister (2004) *Mental Health and Social Exclusion. Social Exclusion Unit Report*. London: The Stationery Office.
Oliver, M. (1990) *The Politics of Disablement*. Basingstoke: Macmillan.
ONS (Office for National Statistics) (2004) *Labour Force Survey*. London: HMSO.
Onyett, S. (2003) *Teamworking in Mental Health*. Basingstoke: Palgrave Macmillan.
Opie, A. (1997) 'Thinking teams thinking clients; issues of discourse and representation in the work of health care teams', *Sociology of Health and Illness*, 19(3): 259–80.
Park, A. (ed.) (2005) *British Social Attitudes. The 22nd Report*. London: Sage.
Parker, I., Georgaca, E., Harper, D., McLaughlin, T. and Stowell-Smith, M. (1995) *Deconstructing Psychopathology*. London: Sage.
Parry-Jones, W. (1972) *The Trade in Lunacy*. London: Routledge.
Payne, M. (2005) *The Origins of Social Work*. Basingstoke: Palgrave Macmillan.
Payne, S. (2000) *Poverty, Social Exclusion and Mental Health: Findings from the 1999 PSE Survey Working Paper No. 15*. Townsend Centre for International Poverty Research, University of Bristol.
Peck, E., Gulliver, P. and Towell, D. (2002) *Modernising Partnerships: an Evaluation of Somerset's Innovations in the Commissioning and Organisation of Mental Health Services – Final Report*. London: Institute of Applied Health and Social Policy, King's College.
Penfold, P.S. and Walker, G.A. (1984) *Women and the Psychiatric Paradox*. Milton Keynes: Open University Press.
Perring, C., Twigg, J. and Atkin, K. (1990) *Families Caring for People Diagnosed as Mentally Ill: the Literature Re-examined*. London: HMSO.
Philo, G. (1996) *Media and Mental Distress*. London: Longman.
Pilgrim, D. and Rogers, A. (1996) 'Two notions of risk in mental health debates', in T. Heller, J. Reynolds, R. Gomm, R. Muston and S. Pattison (eds), *Mental Health Matters. A Reader*. Basingstoke: Macmillan/The Open University.
Pilgrim, D. and Rogers, A. (2005) *A Sociology of Mental Health and Illness*, 3rd edn. Buckingham: Oxford University Press.
Pilgrim, D., Rogers, A. and Tummey, R. (2008) 'The lifespan', in R. Tummey and T. Turner (eds), *Critical Issues in Mental Health*. Basingstoke: Palgrave Macmillan.
Pilkington, N.W. and D'Augelli, A.R. (1995) 'Victimization of lesbian, gay, and bisexual youth in community settings', *Journal of Community Psychology* 23(1): 33–56.
Poole, R. (2006) 'Medical diagnosis of mental illness', in T. Ryan and J. Pritchard (eds), *Good Practice in Adult Mental Health*. London: Jessica Kingsley Publishers.
Porter, R. (1987a) *Mind-forg'd Manacles*. London: Athlone.
Porter, R. (1987b) *A Social History of Madness: Stories of the Insane*. London: Weidenfeld and Nicolson.
Preston, C., Cheater, F., Baker, R. and Hearnshaw, H. (1999) 'Left in limbo: patients' views on care across the primary/secondary interface', *Quality in Health Care*, 8(1): 16–21.
Prime Minister's Strategy Unit (2007) *Building on Progress: Public Services*. London: Prime Minister's Strategy Unit.
Prior, L. (1993) *The Social Organisation of Mental Illness*. London: Sage.
QAA (Quality Assurance Agency for Higher Education) (2008) *Subject Benchmark Statement: Social Work 2008*. Mansfield: QAA.
Read, J. and Baker, S. (1996) *Not Just Sticks and Stones: A Survey of the Stigma, Taboos and Discrimination Experienced by People with Mental Health Problems*. London: MIND.

Reddy, S. (1996) 'Claims to expert knowledge and the subversion of democracy: the triumph of risk over uncertainty', *Economy and Society*, 25(2): 222–54.

Reeves, S., Zwarenstein, M., Goldman, J., Barr, H., Freeth, H., Hammick, M. and Koppel, I. (2008) 'Interprofessional education: effects on professional practice and health care outcomes (Review)', The Cochrane Collaboration. London: Wiley Publishers. www.thecochranelibrary.com

Repper, J., Sayce, L., Strong, S., Willmot, J. and Haines, M. (1997) *Tall Stories from the Back Yard*. London: MIND.

Resisters (2002) *Women Speak Out: Women's Experiences of Using Mental Health Services and Proposals for Change*. Leeds: Resisters.

Rethink (2003) *Who Cares? The Experiences of Mental Health Carers Accessing Services and Information*. Kingston upon Thames: Rethink.

Rethink and EUFAMI and Astra Zeneca (2005) *Putting Mental Health at the Heart of European Union Policy*. Kingston upon Thames: Rethink.

Revill, J. (2006) 'No reguge, no shelter', *The Observer*, 17 September 2006.

Reynolds, S. and Trinder, L. (2000) *Evidence-based Practice: a Critical Approach*. London: Blackwell.

Rivers, I. (2000) 'Long-term consequences of bullying', in C. Neal and D. Davies (eds), *Issues in Therapy with Lesbian, Gay, Bisexual and Transgender Clients*. Buckingham: Open University Press.

Rivers, I. (2001) 'The bullying of sexual minorities at school: its nature and long-term correlates', *Educational and Child Psychology*, 18: 32–46.

Rivett, G. (1997) *From Cradle to Grave*. London: King's Fund.

Rogers and Pilgrim (1996) *Mental Health Policy in Britain*, 1st edn. Basingstoke: Palgrave.

Rogers, A. and Pilgrim, D. (2001) *Mental Health Policy in Britain*, 2nd edn. Basingstoke: Palgrave.

Rogers, A. and Pilgrim, D. (2003) *Mental Health and Inequality*. Basingstoke: Palgrave Macmillan.

Rogers, A., Pilgrim, D. and Lacey, R. (1993) *Experiencing Psychiatry: Users' Views of Services*. London: Macmillan.

Romme, M. and Escher, S. (1993) (eds) *Accepting Voices*. London: MIND.

Rooney, B. (1987) *Racism and Resistance to Change*. Merseyside Area Profile Group/University of Liverpool.

Rose, D. (2001) *Users' Voices: The Perspectives of Mental Health Service Users on Community and Hospital Care*. London: Sainsbury Centre for Mental Health.

Rose, D., Ford, R., Lindley, P. and Gawith, L. (1998) *In Our Experience: User Focused Monitoring of Mental Health Services in Kensington & Chelsea and Westminster Health Authority*. London: Sainsbury Centre for Mental Health.

Rose, N. (1979) 'The psychological complex: mental measurement and social administration', *Ideology and Consciousness*, 5: 5–68.

Rose, N. (1986) 'Law, rights and psychiatry', in P. Miller and N. Rose (eds), *The Power of Psychiatry*. Cambridge: Cambridge University Press.

Russell, D. (1997) *Scenes from Bedlam*. Oxford: Bailliere Tindall.

Ruthen, P. (2006) 'Electroconvulsive therapy (ECT) – the imposition of "truth"?', SCRIPT-Ed, 3(4): 412–36.

Rutter, P. (1995) *Sex in the Forbidden Zone: When Men in Power Abuse Women's Trust*. London: Aquarian.

Sainsbury, R., Irvine, A., Aston, J., Wilson, S., Williams, C. and Sinclair, A. (2008) *Mental Health and Employment*. Research Report No. 513. Norwich: HMSO.

Samele, C., Wallcraft, J., Naylor, C., Keating, F. and Greatley, A. (2007) *Research Priorities for Service User and Carer-Centred Mental Health Services*. London: Sainsbury Centre for Mental Health.

Sartorious, N. (2002) 'Iatrogenic stigma of mental illness: begins with behaviour and attitudes of medical professionals, especially psychiatrists', *British Medical Journal*, 324(7352): 1470–1.

Sayce, L. (2000) *From Psychiatric Patient to Citizen. Overcoming Discrimination and Social Exclusion*. Basingstoke: Macmillan.

Scheff, T. (1966) *Being Mentally Ill: A Sociological Theory*. Chicago: Aldine.

SCIE (Social Care Institute for Excellence) (2006) *Social Work Education Knowledge Review 10. The Learning, Teaching and Assessment of Partnership Work in Social Work Education*. London: Social Care Institute for Excellence.

SCIE (Social Care Institute for Excellence) (2008) *Research Briefing 26. Mental Health and Social Work*. London: SCIE.

SCMH (Sainsbury Centre for Mental Health) (1999) *The National Service Framework for Mental Health: an Executive Briefing*. London: SCMH.

SCMH (Sainsbury Centre for Mental Health) (2000a) *The Capable Practitioner Framework*. London: SCMH.

SCMH (Sainsbury Centre for Mental Health) (2000b) *Taking your Partners*. London: SCMH.

SCMH (Sainsbury Centre for Mental Health) (2002) *Breaking the Circles of Fear Between Mental Health Services and African and Caribbean Communities*. London: SCMH.

SCMH (Sainsbury Centre for Mental Health) (2006) *The Future of Mental Health: a Vision for 2015*. London: SCMH.

Scobie, S., Minghella, E., Dale, C., Thomson, R., Lelliott, P. and Hill, K. (2006) With Safety in Mind: *Mental Health Services and Patient Safety*. London: National Patient Safety Agency.

Scott, S. and Williams, J. (2001) *Report on Department of Health User/Survivor Consultation Day*. Canterbury: Tizard Centre, University of Kent.

Scottish Executive (2002) *Choose Life: A National Strategy and Action Plan to Prevent Suicide in Scotland*. Edinburgh: Scottish Executive.

Scull, A. (1977) *Decarceration. Community Treatment and the Deviant. A Radical View*. New Jersey: Prentice Hall.

Scull, A. (1979) *Museums of Madness*. London: Penguin.

Scull, A. (1981) *Madhouses, Mad Doctors and Madmen*. London: Athlone Press.

Scull, A. (1993) *The Most Solitary of Afflictions*. London: Yale University Press.

Scull, A. (1996) 'Asylums, utopias and realities', in D. Tomlinson and J. Carrier (eds), *Asylum in the Community*. London: Routledge.

Seebohm, R. (1968) *Report of the Committee on Local Authority and Allied Personal Social Services*. London: HMSO.

Sharkey, P. (2007) *The Essentials of Community Care*, 2nd edn. Basingstoke: Palgrave Macmillan.

Sheppard, M. (1991) 'General practice, social work and mental health sections: the social control of women', *British Journal of Social Work*, 21: 663–83.

Sheppard, M. (2002) 'Mental health and social justice: gender, race and psychological consequences of unfairness', *British Journal of Social Work*, 32: 779–97.

Shorter, E. (1997) *A History of Psychiatry*. London: John Wiley & Sons.

Showalter, E. (1987) *The Female Malady: Women, Madness and English Culture, 1830–1980*. London: Virago.

Simoni-Wastila, L. (2000) 'The use of abusable prescription drugs: the role of gender', *Journal of Women's Health and Gender Based Medicine*, 9: 289–97.

Simpson, T. (2004) *Doorways in the Night: Stories from the Threshold of Recovery*. Leeds: Local Voices.

Singleton, N., Bumpstead, R., O'Brian, M., Lee, A. and Meltzer, H. (2001) *Psychiatric Morbidity Among Adults Living in Private Households, 2000*. London: HMSO.

Singleton, N., Maung, N.A., Cowie, A., Sparks, J., Bumpstead, R. and Meltzer, H. (2002) *Mental Health of Carers*. London: HMSO.

Skultans, V. (1979) *English Madness. Ideas on Insanity 1580–1890*. London: RKP.

SPN (Social Perspectives Network) (2003a) *SPN Paper 3. Start Making Sense … Developing Social Models to Understand and Work with Mental Distress*. London: Social Perspectives Network.

SPN (Social Perspectives Network) (2003b) *SPN Paper 2. What is the Knowledge Base and Where Does it Come From?* London: Social Perspectives Network.

SPN (Social Perspectives Network) (2004) *SPN Paper 6. Integration of Health and Social Care: Promoting Social Care Perspectives within Integrated Mental Health Services*. London: Social Perspectives Network.

SPN (Social Perspectives Network) (2005) *SPN Paper 7. Women and Mental Health: Turning Rhetoric into Reality – Sharing Practice Perspectives and Strategies for Action on Women's Mental Health*. London: Social Perspectives Network.

SPN (Social Perspectives Network) (2007) *Whose Recovery is it Anyway?* London: Social Perspectives Network.

SPN (Social Perspectives Network) (2008) *Personalisation: Steps on the Journey*, http://www.spn.org.uk/index.php?id=1200 (accessed 19 December 2008).

Spurrell, M., Hatfield, B. and Perry, A. (2003) 'Characteristics of patients presenting for emergency psychiatric assessment at an English hospital', *Psychiatric Services*, 54(2): 240–5.

Stark, S., Skidmore, D., Warne, T. and Stronach, I. (2002) 'A survey of "teamwork" in mental health: is it achievable in practice?', *British Journal of Nursing*, 11(3): 178–86.

Stonewall (2007) *Education for All. Research. Facts and Figures. Mental Health*. London: Stonewall.

SWAP (The Social Policy and Social Work Subject Centre of the Higher Education Academy) and MHHE (The Mental Health in Higher Education Project) (2007) *Towards A New Vision for Mental Health Education: Developments at Qualification and Post-Qualification Levels*. University of Birmingham: MHHE/HEA, www.mhhe.heacademy.ac.uk/silo/files/social-work-event-reportjun07towards-a-new-vision.doc (accessed 8 May 2009).

Szasz, T.S. (1961) *The Myth of Mental Illness*. New York: Hoeber-Harper.

Taylor, R. (1994/95) 'Alienation and integration in mental health policy', *Critical Social Policy*, 42(14): 81–90.

Taylor, P. and Gunn, J. (1999) 'Homicides by people with mental illness: myth and reality', *British Journal of Psychiatry*, 174: 9–14.

Tew, J. (2002) 'Going social: championing a holistic model of mental distress within professional education', *Social Work Education*, 21(2): 143–55.

Tew, J. (2003) 'Core themes for social models of mental distress', in Social Perspectives Network *SPN Paper 3. Start Making Sense … Developing Social Models to Understand and Work with Mental Distress*. London: Social Perspectives Network.

Tew, J. (ed.) (2005) *Social Perspectives in Mental Health. Developing Social Models to Understand and Work with Mental Distress*. London: Jessica Kingsley Publishers.

Thomas, P. (1997) *The Dialectics of Schizophrenia*. London: Free Association Books.

Thompson, N. (2006) *Anti-discriminatory Practice*, 4th edn. Basingstoke: Palgrave Macmillan.

Thornicroft, G., Rose, D., Kassam, A. and Sartorious, N. (2007) 'Stigma: ignorance, prejudice or discrimination?', *British Journal of Psychiatry*, 190: 192–3.

Thornicroft, G. (2006) *Shunned: Discrimination Against People with Mental Illness.* Oxford: Oxford University Press.

Thornicroft, G., Rose, D., Huxley, P., Dale, G. and Wykes, T. (2002) 'What are the research priorities of mental health service users?', *Journal of Mental Health*, 11: 1–5.

Timimi, S. (2005) *Naughty Boys. Anti-social Behaviour, ADHD and the Role of Culture.* Basingstoke: Palgrave Macmillan.

Titmuss, R. (1968) *Commitment to Welfare.* London: Allen & Unwin.

TNS (Taylor Nelson Sofres) (2007) *Attitudes to Mental Illness 2007.* London: CSIP/Shift.

Torrey, E.F. (2003) *The Invisible Plague.* New Jersey: Rutgers University Press.

TOPSS England (Training Organisation for Personal Social Services in England) (2002) *The National Occupational Standards for Social Work.* Leeds: TOPSS England.

Turner, E.H., Matthews, A.M., Linardatos, B.S., Tell, R.A. and Rosenthal, R. (2008) 'Selective publication of antidepressant trials and its influence on apparent efficiency', *New England Journal of Medicine*, 358(3): 252–60.

Ungerson, C. (1987) *Policy is Personal: Sex, Gender and Informal Care.* London: Routledge.

Ussher, J.M. (1991) *Women's Madness: Misogyny or Mental Illness?* Hemel Hempstead: Harvester Wheatsheaf.

Vassilev, I. and Pilgrim, D. (2007) 'Risk, trust and the myth of mental health services', *Journal of Mental Health*, 16(3): 347–57.

Wallcraft, J. and Bryant, M. (2003) *The Mental Health Service User Movement in England.* London: Sainsbury Centre for Mental Health.

Walls, P. and Sashidharan S.P. (2003) *Real Voices: Survey Findings from a Series of Community Consultation Events Involving Black and Minority Ethnic Groups in England.* London: Department of Health.

Walton, R.G. (1975) *Women and Social Work.* London: RKP.

Warner, J., McKeown, E., Griffin, M., Johnson, K., Ramsay, A., Cort, C. and King, M. (2004) 'Rates predictors of mental illness in gay men, lesbians and bisexual men and women', *British Journal of Psychiatry*, 185: 479–85.

Webb, S. (2006) *Social Work in a Risk Society. Social and Political Perspectives.* Basingstoke: Palgrave Macmillan.

Webber, M. (2008) *Evidence-based Policy and Practice in Mental Health Social Work.* Exeter: Learning Matters.

Wetzel, J.W. (2000) 'Women and mental health: a global perspective', *International Social Work*, 34(2): 205–15.

Whittington, C. (2003) *Learning for Collaborative Practice with Other Professions and Agencies.* London: Department of Health.

WHO (World Health Organization) (1946) *Constitution.* New York: WHO.

WHO (World Health Organization) (1992) *Tenth Revision of the International Classification of Diseases and Related Health Problems (ICD–10).* Geneva: WHO.

WHO (World Health Organization) (1995) *Bridging the Gaps.* Geneva: WHO.

WHO (World Health Organization) (2000) *Women's Mental Health: an Evidence Based Review.* Geneva: WHO.

WHO (World Health Organization) (2001a) *Strengthening Mental Health Promotion (Factsheet no. 220).* Geneva: WHO.

WHO (World Health Organization) (2001b) *Fifty-fourth World Health Assembly. Round Tables: Mental Health. Report by the Secretariat.* Geneva: WHO.

WHO (World Health Organization) (2001c) *Gender Disparities in Mental Health.* Geneva: WHO.

WHO (World Health Organization) (2002) *Gender and Mental Health.* Geneva: WHO.

WHO (World Health Organization) (2004) *Prevention of Mental Disorders. Effective Interventions and Policy Options, Summary Report*. Geneva: WHO.

WHO (World Health Organization) (2007) *Mental Health*, www.who.int/topics/mental_health/en/ (accessed 31 October 2007).

WHO (World Health Organization) (2008) *Policies and Practices for Mental Health in Europe*. Geneva: WHO.

Williams, J. (1999) 'Social inequalities and mental health', in C. Newnes, G. Holmes and C. Dunn (eds), *This is Madness: a Critical Look at Psychiatry and the Future of Mental Health Services*. Ross on Wye: PCCS Books.

Williams, B., Copestake, P., Eversley, J. and Stafford, B. (2008) *Experiences and Expectations of Disabled People*. London: Office for Disability Issues.

Wood, D. (1993) *The Power of Words. Uses and Abuses of Talking Treatments*. London: MIND.

World Psychiatric Association (2001) *The WPA Global Programme to Reduce the Stigma and Discrimination because of Schizophrenia – an Interim Report 2001*. Geneva: World Psychiatric Association.

Younghusband, E. (1978) *Social Work in Britain: 1950–1975, Vols 1 and 2*. London: Allen & Unwin.

INDEX

NOTE: Page numbers in **bold type** refer to boxes

abuse of women, 115, 116
actuarialism, 77
admissions, 63, 69–72, 78–80
age, 120–1
ageism, **120**
akathesia, 92
Alaszewski, A., 77
American Psychiatric Association, 16
anti-depressants, 91, 100–1
anti-discrimination policy, **110**, 112, 114, 116, 118
anti-oppressive theory and practice, 108–21
anti-psychiatry movement, 122
anti-psychotic medication, 91–2
Appleby, L., 57, 76
Approved Clinician (AC), 66
Approved Mental Health Practitioner (AMHP), 66, 73–4, 139–40
Approved Social Worker (ASW), 35, 66, 73, 139–40
Arskey, H., 42
assessments, 17–20, 43, 45–6, 57–8
asylums, 28–30
attitudes to mental distress, 8–14, 104, 111–14, 115–16, 117–18, 146
 see also discrimination; moral panics
Audit Commission, 139

Baker, S., 12, 116
Bamford, T., 20
Barclay Committee, 35
Barham, P., 48
Barnes, M., 104
Bartlett, P., 25, 27, 59
Bebbington, P., 115
behaviour therapy, 94
Bennett Inquiry, 113, 114
Bentall, R., 16
Beresford, P., 58–9, 104, 124
Berger, J., 109
Best Interests Assessor (BIA), 68
Bethlem Royal Hospital (Bedlam), 26–7, 122
Beveridge Report, 32
biological approaches, 89–93
 see also medical model
Black and Minority Ethnic Mental Health Programme, 114
Boardman, J., 59

Bogg, D., 139
Borrill, C.S., 138
Bournewood judgement, 68
Bowl, R., 104
Bracken, P., 13, 17, 19, 96
Bradshaw, J., 42
Braithwaite, T., 144
Brammer, A., 80–1
Breggin, P., 90
Brewis, R., 57
Brown, G.W., 96
Brown, J., 42
Brown, P., 28
budgets, 45, 56–7, 58–9, **131**
Busfield, J., 36
Butterfield, P., 90
Bynum, W.F., 29
Bytheway, B., 120

Campbell, P., 123
care management approach, 37–8, 45, 46, 52, 79, 133
Care Programme Approach (CPA), 46, 52–6, 57, 133
Care Quality Commission, 69
Care Trusts, 131
carers, 42–4
 needs of, 18, 43, 142, 143–5
 perspectives of, 102, 103–4, 143
 policy relating to, 43–4
Carers and Disabled Children Act (2000), 43
Carers (Equal Opportunities) Act (2004), 43–4
Carers (Recognition and Services) Act (1996), 18, 43
Carr, S., 118
Castel, R., 78
CCTA (Creating Capable Teams Approach), 135
Central Council for Education and Training in Social Work (CCETSW), 34
Certificate of Qualification in Social Work (CQSW), 34
Chaplin, R., 14
charity, 32
Charlton, B.G., 92–3
child protection, 131–2
children, and mental distress, 120
choice, 57, 58

Clarke, J., 32, 37
class, 111–12
Clements, J., 48
CMHTs (Community Mental Health Teams), 52, 134, 139
Cochrane, A., 37
Code of Practice: Mental Health Act 1983 (DH), 64–5
Codes of Practice for Social Care Workers and Employers (GSCC), 83
cognitive behaviour therapy (CBT), 94, 95–6
collaboration *see* integrated working; interprofessional working
commodification of welfare, 45
community care
 in 1990s, 44–7
 care programme approach, 46, 52–6, 57, 133
 compulsory powers, 72–3
 defining, 42
 evaluating, 53–5, 59
 history, 25
 media and moral panics, 47–8
 personalization agenda and future, 56–9
 policy, 49–52
 providers, 42–4
 transition to, 34, 35–8
Community Mental Health Teams (CMHTs), 52, 134, 139
Community Treatment Order (CTO), 73, 79–80
compulsory admission, 63, 78–80
 sectioning, 69–72
compulsory assessments, 18
compulsory powers in community, 72–3
consent, 89, 90
consumerist discourse, 123–4
Cooper, A., 99
Coppock, V., 115, 121
County Asylums Act (1808), 28
CPA *see* Care Programme Approach
CQSW (Certificate of Qualification in Social Work), 34
Creating Capable Teams Approach (CCTA), 135
Crossley, N., 122
CSIP (Care Services Improvement Partnership), 147
CTO *see* Community Treatment Order
cultural context of discrimination, 108–9
cultural diversity, 112

Danbury, H., 34
dangerousness, 47, 77–8
D'Augelli, A.R., 118
Davies, M., 35
Davis, A., 144, 145
De Swaan, A., 18

deinstitutionalization, 35–7, 48
dementia, 121
Department of Health (DH), 9, 97, 116
 policy *see* legislation and policy
depression, 96, 121
 medication for, 91, 100–1
Deprivation of Liberty Safeguards (DoLS), 64, 68
diagnosis, 13, 15–17
Diagnostic and Statistical Manual of Mental Disorders (DSM), 15, 16, 118
disability, 119–20
Disability Discrimination Act (2005), 112
Disability Equality Duty (2006), 112
disablism, **119**
discrimination
 fighting, 122–5
 forms of, 13–14, 110–21
 theorizing, 108–10
diversity issues, 108–21
DoLS (Deprivation of Liberty Safeguards), 64, 68
Donnelly, M., 28, 29
Double, D.B., 15, 16, 19
Doyal, L., 115
drug companies, 100–1
drug treatments, 36, 79, 91–2, 100–1, 116
DSM (*Diagnostic and Statistical Manual of Mental Disorders*), 15, 16, 118
Duggan, M., 99, 103, 105
Dunn, S., 12
Dustin, D., 45

economic factors, in deinstitutionalization, 36
education and training, 34, 135–7
electroconvulsive therapy (ECT), 89–91, 116
empowerment, 123–4
 see also choice
Engels, F., 32
ethics, 82–4
 see also values
European Court of Human Rights, 80–1
evidence, and power dynamics, 100–1, 102–3
evidence-based practice (EBP), 101–3
 and user perspectives, 102, 103–4

Faulkner, A., 90, 104
Fennell, P., 31, 89
Fernando, S., 112
Fook, J., 78
formal patients, 63
Foster, J., 99, 137, 139, 143
Foucault, M., 10, 29, 102
Francis, E., 47
Freud, S., 93
Frosh, S., 117
Future Vision Coalition, 146, 148

Index

gender, 43, 91, 115–17
Gender Equality Duty, 116
General Social Care Council (GSCC), 83
Gibbons, J., 28
Glendinning, C., 42
Glennerster, H., 46
Goffman, E., 18
Griffiths Report, 37
guardianship, 72

Hannigan, B., 46
Harris, J., 38, 45
Harris, T., 96
Hawton, K., 117
Health Act (1999), 131
health professionals
  attitudes and assumptions of, 13–14, 97
  power of, 27
  relationship with social workers, 139–40
  roles, 66–7
  see also mental health professionals
Healthcare Commission, 54
Hearing Voices Network, 99
Helm, A., 98
heterosexism, **117**, 118
holistic approach to assessment, 19–20
homophobia, **117**, 118
hospital managers, 67
human rights, 123–4
Human Rights Act (1998), 80–2
human rights based practice, 124–5
Human Rights Insight Project, 81
Huxley, P., 139

iatrogenic effects, 91–2
ICD (*International Statistical Classification of Diseases and Related Problems*), 15, 118
images of mental distress, 11–14
impairment, **119**
Independent Mental Health Advocates (IMHAs), 68
individual budgets, 56–7, 58–9
inequality, 11, 97, 146
  fighting, 122–5
  forms of, 110–21
  theorizing, 108–10
informal patients, 63
institutional care, 26–7, 36
  asylums, 28–30
  madhouses, 27–8
  see also deinstitutionalization
institutional racism, **113**, 114
institutional sexism, 115
integrated working, 52, 58, 129–30, 131–2, 142–5
interdisciplinary working, **20–1**, 46

International Statistical Classification of Diseases and Related Problems (ICD), 15, 118
interprofessional education and training, 135–7
interprofessional working, 128–9
  policy, 130–5
  research findings, 137–9
  social work contribution, 140, **141–2**
  tensions in, 139–40
  terminology, 129–30, 136
  user and carer needs, 142–5
  workforce reform, 134–5
  see also integrated working; interdisciplinary working
IPE (interprofessional education), 136
Irvine, E., 33

Ioannides, D., 124
Jodelet, D., 10–11
Johns, R., 82
Johnstone, L., 90–1
Jones, C., 99
Jones, K., 25, 26, 27, 29, 30, 31, 32, 33, 34, 38, 42
Jordan, B., 31

Kemshall, H., 77, 79
Kendall, T., 100
Kirsch, I., 91

Laming Report, 136
Langan, J., 37
Langan, M., 34, 35
lead commissioning, **131**
legislation and policy
  anti-discrimination, **110**, 112, 114, 116, 118
  on carers, 43–4
  on community care, 36–7, 44–7, 49–52
  on compulsory detention and treatment, 63, 69–72, 78–80
  compulsory powers in community, 72–3
  defining mental disorder, 65–6
  and development of social work, 31–5
  evolving, 47–8, 63
  human rights, 80–2
  impact and future of, 56–9, 146, 148
  impact of users on, 123–4
  implementation, 63
  on institutional care, 26–31
  on interprofessional working, 130–5
  statutory context for practice, 63–4
  theorizing risk, 75–8
  see also Mental Health Act
Lewis, J., 46

Local Authority Social Services Act (1970), 34
Local Implementation Teams (LITs), 53
Lunacy Act (1845), 28
Lunacy Act (1890), 30
Lupton, D., 77–8

McCrae, N., 134
McDonaldisation of social work, 45
McFarlane, L., 118
McKay, D., 14
McKenna, H., 103
MacKenzie, C., 27
McKnight, J., 97
McLaughlin, K., 79
McLean, R., 140
Macmillan Commission (1926), 31
MacPherson, J., 12
Macpherson Report, 113, 114
madhouse system, 27–8
Malek, M., 121
managerialism, 45, 103, 123–4
Mandelstam, M., 53, 59
Means, R., 37
media, 11–12, 47–8
medical model, 15–16, 18, 19, 92–3, 105, 119, 120–1, 146
  see also biological approach
medical profession see health professionals
medication see drug treatments
Meltzer, H., 111
men, and mental distress, 117
mental disorder, legal definition, 65–6
mental distress
  attitudes to, 8–14, 104, 111–14, 115–16, 117–18, 146
  defining, 7–8, 65–6, 112
  and forms of inequality, 110–21
  images and representations of, 11–14
  prevalence, 10, 28, 29
  terminology of, 12, 15
  theories of, 15–17
  treatment of see treatment
mental health
  defining, 7–8, 112
  theorising, 15–17
Mental Health Act (1959), 33–4
Mental Health Act (1983), 18, 35, 63–5
  key roles under, 66–9, 73–4
  powers in community under, 72–3
  sectioning process, 69–72
Mental Health Act (2007), 8, 64, 66
  key roles under, 66–9, 73–4
  powers in community under, 73
Mental Health Act Commission (MHAC), 69, 90
Mental Health Alliance, 64
Mental Health Care Trusts, 134

Mental Health Foundation, 13, 90, 121
Mental Health (Patients in the Community) Act (1995), 48
mental health policy see legislation and policy
Mental Health Policy Implementation Guide, 134
mental health professionals
  attitudes to users, 13–14, 97, 104
  education and training, 34, 135–7
  key roles, 66–9
  power of, 27, 124
  tension between, 139–40
  workforce reform, 134–5
  see also interprofessional working; professional practice; social workers
Mental Health Review Tribunal (MHRT), 68
mental health services
  care programme approach, 46, 52–6, 57, 133
  New Labour's modernization of, 49–52, 54, 130–1, 132–5
  see also users
mental health system
  history of
    asylums, 28–30
    institutional care, 26–7
    madhouses, 27–8
    mental hospitals, 30–1
    pre-history, 25
    social work practice, 31–5
    transition to community, 35–8
mental health treatments see treatment
mental hospitals, establishment of, 30–1
mental illness see mental distress
Mental Patients' Union, 122–3
Mental Treatment Act (1930), 31
Mental Welfare Officers, 33–4
MHAC (Mental Health Act Commission), 69
MHRT (Mental Health Review Tribunal), 68
Milne, A., 115
MIND, 10, 12, 17, 92, 93, 98, 117, 121
modernization agenda, 49–52, 54, 130–1, 132–5
Moncrieff, J., 100
moral panics, 47–8
Morris, J., 119, 120
Muijen, , M., 46, 48
multi-disciplinary working, 46, 129
  see also integrated working; interprofessional working
multiprofessional education, 136
Murphy, E., 29

National Carers Strategy (1998), 43
National Carers Strategy (2008), **44**
National Framework of Values for Mental Health, 83–4

Index

National Institute for Health and Clinical Excellence (NICE), 89–90
National Institute for Mental Health in England (NIMHE), **83–4**, 114, 140, 147
National Service Framework for Mental Health (NSFMH), 19, 43, **49–51**, 133–4, 146
nearest relative (NR), 67
needs of carers, 18, 43, 142, 143–5
needs-led provision, 45–6
New Labour policy, 49–52, 54, 130–4
New Ways of Working (NWW) programme, 135
Newnes, C., 24
NHS, establishment of, 32–3
NHS and Community Care Act (1990), 18, 37, 45, 123, 130
NHS Plan, 51, 131
NICE (National Institute for Health and Clinical Excellence), 89–90
NIMHE (National Institute for Mental Health in England), **83–4**, 114, 140, 147
Norman, I.J., 138
NSFMH *see National Service Framework for Mental Health*
NWW (New Ways of Working) programme, 135

older people, 121
Oliver, M., 119
oppression *see* discrimination

Park, A., 118
Parker, I., 7
Parry-Jones, W., 27
partnership, 20, 52, 130
  see also integrated working
Partnership Trusts, 134
patriarchy, **115**
Payne, S., 32, 45, 111
PCS analysis, 8–9, 19, 108–10, 114
Peck, E., 138
person-centred therapy, 95
personal level of discrimination, 108
personalization agenda, 56–8, 124
Philo, G., 12
Pilgrim, D., 7, 18, 19, 27, 30, 31, 37, 47, 48, 63, 77, 78, 80, 93, 120
Pilkington, N.W., 118
Pinel P., 28
policy *see* legislation and policy
Poole, R., 16
pooled budgets, **131**
Porter, R., 25, 28, 29, 122
poverty, 111, 115
power dynamics, in EBP, 100–1, 102–3
principles, underlying MHA, **65**
professional practice
  evidence-based, 101–4
  human rights based, 124–5

professional practice *cont.*
  statutory context, 63–4
  see also social work
professionals *see* mental health professionals
psychiatric diagnosis, 13, 15–17
psychiatric social work (PSW), 32, 33
psychiatry, 15, 24, 25
  anti-psychiatry movement, 122
  and drug companies, 100–1
psychodynamic therapy, 93–4
psychological approaches, 93–6
psychotherapy, 36

race and ethnicity, 47, 112–14
racism, 112–13, 114
Read, J., 116
recovery agenda, 97–100
Reddy, S., 78
Reeves, S., 136
Reissman, K., 54
representations of mental distress, 11–14
research
  evidence-based practice, 101–3
  power dynamics in, 100–1, 102–3
  user perspectives in, 103–4
Responsible Clinician (RC), 67
Rethink, 42
Revill, J., 54
risk, theorizing, 75–8
risk assessment, 47
risk management, 75–7
Rivers, I., 118
Rivett, G., 33
Rogers, A., 7, 17, 18, 19, 27, 30, 31, 37, 47, 48, 63, 93, 120
Rose, D., 104
Russell, D., 26, 27

Sainsbury, R., 111
Sartorious, N., 13
Sashidharan, S.P., 113
Sayce, L., 11, 111, 119
Scheff, T., 18
SCIE (Social Care Institute for Excellence), 130, 142, 147
Scobie, S., 116
Scott, S., 116
SCT (Supervised Community Treatment), 73
Scull, A., 25, 27, 28, 29, 36
sectioning, 63, 69–72
Seebohm Report, 34
sexism, **115**
sexual orientation, 117–19
shared approach, 58
  see also integrated working
Sharkey, P., 42, 54, 77
Sheldon, K., 13

Shorter, E., 25, 29
Simoni-Wastila, L., 116
Singleton, N., 10
Skultans, V., 25
Smith, R., 37
Smyth, M., 17, 19
social class, 111–12
social deprivation, 31–2
Social Exclusion Unit, 112
social model, 16–17, 19–20, 96–7, **99–100**, 119, 140, 146–7
social work
    contribution of, **20–1**, 140, **141–2**
    critical perspectives in, 147
    development, 31–5
    key elements, 147–8
social workers
    attitudes to users, 97
    changing role of, 37–8, 66
    in CMHTs, 52, 134
    relationship with health professionals, 139–40
    valued by users and carers, 142–3
    see also mental health professionals
SPN (Social Perspectives Network), 21, 142
Spurrell, M., 117
Stark, S., 138–9
Steinberg, D. 120
stereotypes, 11–13, 112–14, 115–16, 117, 121
stigma, 12–14, 111–12
Stonewall, 118
structural level of discrimination, 109
suicide, 117, 118
Supervised Community Treatment (SCT), 73
supervision registers, 48
Szasz, T.S., 29

talking therapies *see* psychological approaches
tardive dyskinesia, 92
Ten Essential Shared Capabilities, 137
Tew, J., 17, 20, 92, 97, 98, 99
therapeutic communities, 36
Thomas, P., 104
Thompson, N., 8, 19, 108–10, 114
Thornicroft, G., 14
Three Keys to a Shared Approach in Mental Health Assessment, 57–8
Timimi, S., 121
Titmuss, R., 33

Torrey, E.F., 28
treatment
    biological approaches, 89–93
    consent to, 89, 90
    as contested arena, 88–9
    early approaches, 25
    psychological approaches, 93–6
    social approaches, 96–7
    see also recovery agenda
Tuke, W., 27–8
Tummey, R., 120
Turner, E.H., 100–1

user movements, 122–4
user-centred practice, 21
User-Focused Monitoring (UFM), 104
users
    choice and empowerment of, 57, 58, 123–4
    needs of, 142–3, 144–5
    perspectives of, 17, 102, 103–4, 146, 148
    and recovery agenda, 98–9

values, 82–4, 102, 147
Vassilev, I., 77, 78, 80
violence, 11–12, 115
voluntary admission, 63

Walker, A., 54
Walls, P., 113
Walton, R.G., 33
Warner, J., 118
Webb, S., 77, 79
Webber, M., 139
welfare state, 32–3
Wetzel, J.W., 115
Whittington, C., 129
WHO (World Health Organisation), 8, 13, 59, 101, 111, 115, 117
Williams, B., 111, 112
Williams, J., 97, 115, 116
women
    as carers, 43
    and mental distress, 91, 115–17
Women's Mental Health Strategy, 116
workforce reform, 134–5
Wright, D., 25, 27, 59

Younghusband, E., 33, 34